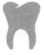

TEETH
AREN'T JUST FOR
SMILING

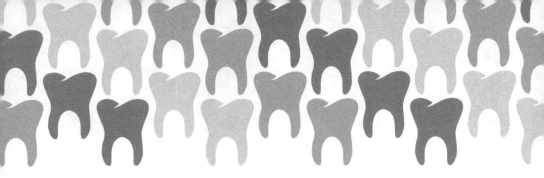

DR. BRETT LANGSTON

TEETH AREN'T JUST FOR SMILING

ORAL CARE AND ITS IMPACT ON THE WHOLE BODY

Advantage | Books

Published by Advantage Books, Charleston, South Carolina.
An imprint of Advantage Media.

ADVANTAGE is a registered trademark, and the Advantage colophon is a trademark of Advantage Media Group, Inc.

Printed in the United States of America.

10 9 8 7 6 5 4 3 2 1

ISBN: 978-1-64225-765-6 (Paperback)
ISBN: 978-1-64225-764-9 (eBook)

LCCN: 2023904553

Book design by Analisa Smith.

This publication is designed to provide accurate and authoritative information in regard to the subject matter covered. It is sold with the understanding that the publisher is not engaged in rendering legal, accounting, or other professional services. If legal advice or other expert assistance is required, the services of a competent professional person should be sought.

Advantage Books is an imprint of Advantage Media Group. Advantage Media helps busy entrepreneurs, CEOs, and leaders write and publish a book to grow their business and become the authority in their field. Advantage authors comprise an exclusive community of industry professionals, idea-makers, and thought leaders. For more information go to **advantagemedia.com**.

I would like to dedicate this book to my amazing wife and soulmate, Lyndsay. She has been with me on my whole journey—from when I was a high schooler who only knew he wanted to be in medicine; through college, where she helped guide my attention to dentistry; and then through dental school and both our residencies, where she was my rock and motivation to keep pushing. My favorite dental cases are those I get to do with her.

I also want to dedicate this book to our fantastic children, Alexis, Bella, and Knox. We are so blessed to have you in our lives, and every day I strive to make you as proud of your dad as I am proud of each one of you!

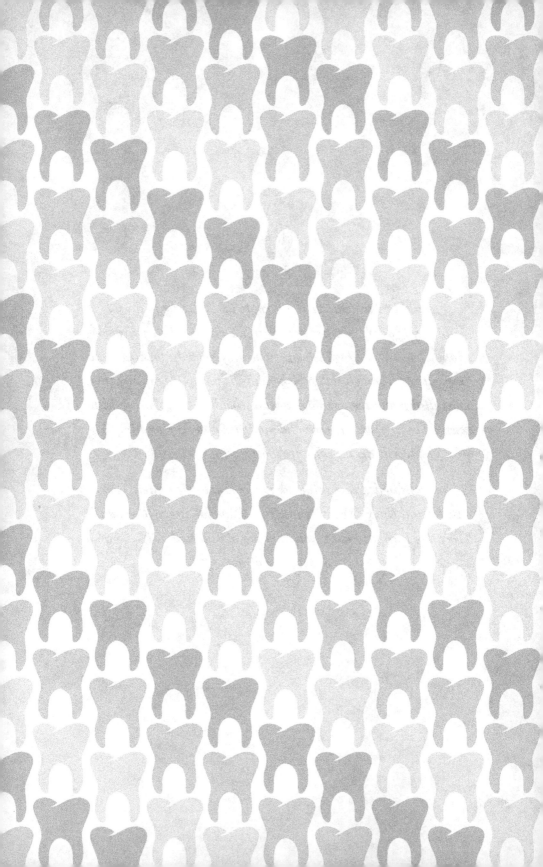

CONTENTS

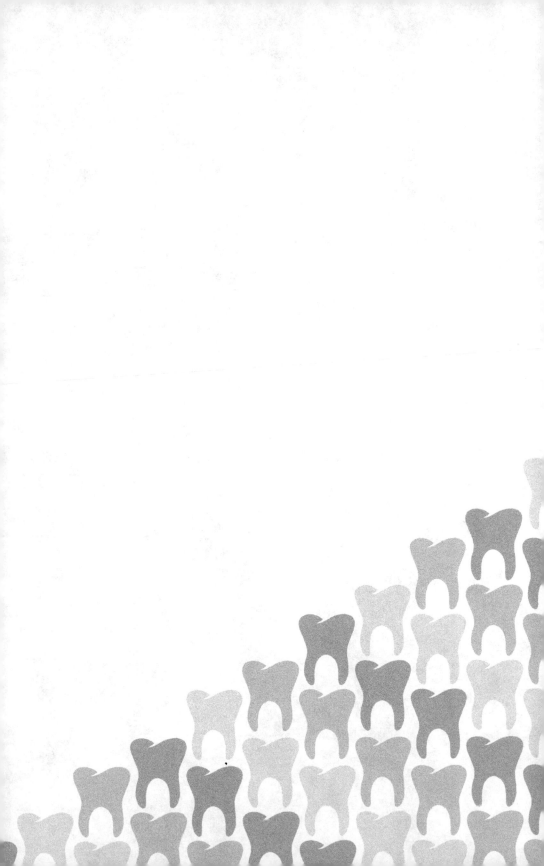

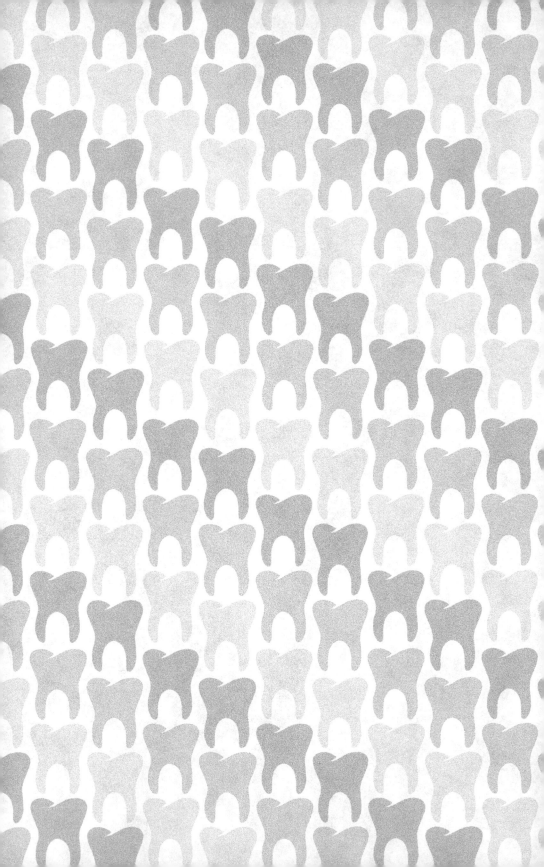

ACKNOWLEDGMENTS

I would like to acknowledge first of all my family—they are the reason I get up every day and cause the beating of my heart every waking moment. I cherish every second I have with them, and they are my most prized possessions.

I also need to show my appreciation to my mom and dad and my sister Amanda, who instilled in me a purpose and a mantra to achieve and make the world a better place. Their constant love and support has kept me grounded and given me the self-confidence to handle any situation. Any great writing genes are a direct blessing from my best-selling-author father, and I appreciate his tutelage and guidance in the literary world. This continued support and all the love from my wife and children empower me to be the person I have become.

I would also like to acknowledge all the wonderful educators who have helped grow my knowledge and guided me on this journey. I have had so many teachers and mentors who helped me focus my energy and attention into a positive force; they have truly pulled the best out of me and allowed me to share my abilities with the world.

I also want to recognize and share the true secret to my success: my dental team. I have found that by surrounding myself with incredible people, I am able to raise my ability to really make a difference in the lives of those I encounter. From my marvelous leadership team that keeps me on track and handles so many things that I can't even begin to thank them for, all the way to how everyone who works with me on a daily basis helps me succeed, I am so fortunate to have such a motivated team to work with.

Lastly, I want to thank God. I have been blessed beyond my wildest imagination, and I know that nothing is impossible with God on my side. I also want to acknowledge my patron saint, Saint Philip Neri; he considered a cheerful temper to be more Christian than a melancholy one and carried this spirit into his whole life: "A joyful heart is more easily made perfect than a downcast one." My biggest hope is that everyone I meet feels his presence in me and is motivated to grow their spiritual strength as mine has grown.

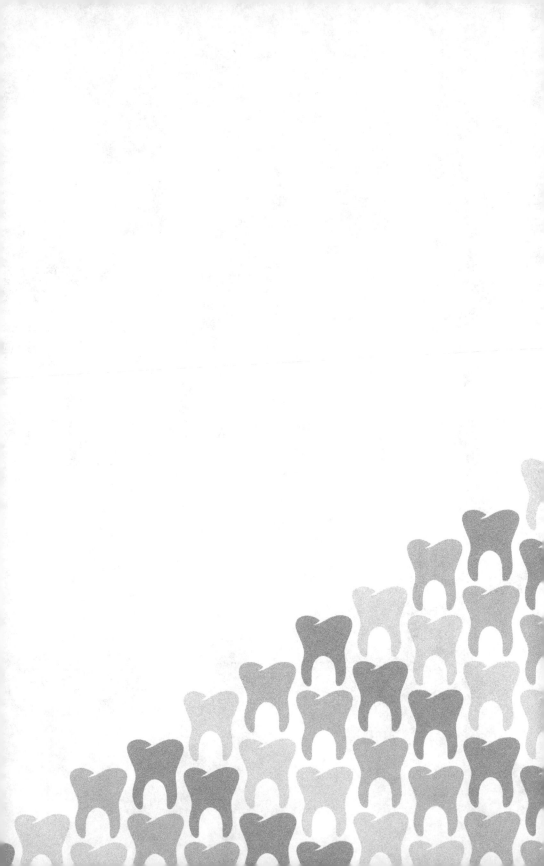

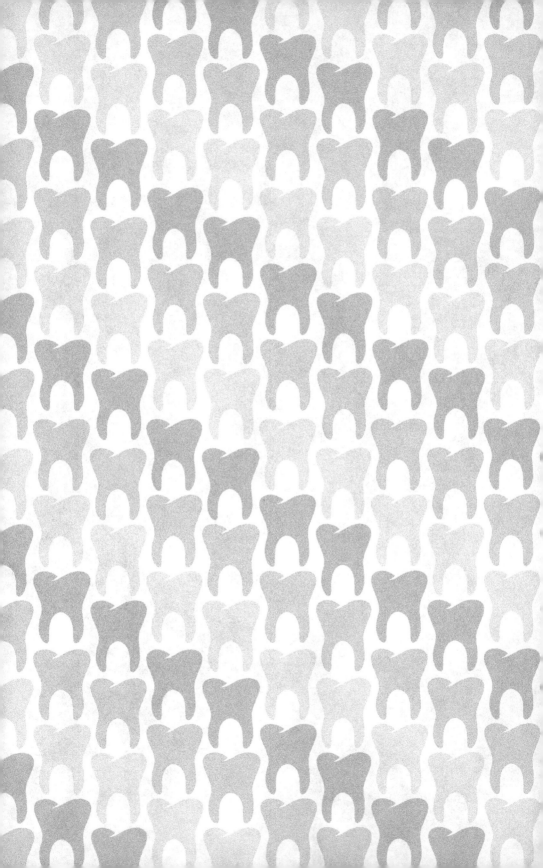

INTRODUCTION

Since prehistoric times, when the first caveman broke off a tooth gnawing on an antelope bone, people have been trying to figure out ways to replace or repair missing and broken teeth. Ancient civilizations tried everything from gold wire to bits of shell or bamboo to put things right. These are the humble beginnings of the dental specialty of prosthodontics, the practice of rehabilitating and maintaining oral function. Fortunately for modern humans, prosthodontics has benefitted from enormous strides in technology, especially in the past decade or so, and we can happily leave ivory and stone tooth replacements in the history books.

I have always loved technology, and as a young man I envisioned a future for myself that included helping people. I thought about becoming an emergency room doctor and saw myself on the front lines at the ER making life-changing decisions in a fast-paced environment, working with the latest in medical technology. But I also dreamed of life as a family man and worried that the demands of the medical profession would compromise that dream. Meeting my wife, Lyndsay, led me on the path that took me to where I am today.

I started college as a premed student, and Lyndsay, who always wanted to be a dentist herself, encouraged me to spend time with both doctors and dentists to get a feel for both professions. After doing so, I realized that dentists could have just as big an impact on people's lives as doctors. My own life was certainly improved by the dental care I received.

As a child, I went for regular checkups and wore braces, but I still had spaces between my teeth that made me feel self-conscious. My dentist built up my teeth using filling material, and the result was a smile that gave me confidence and made me feel good about myself. My own personal experience continued to lurk in the back of my mind, and after recalling how it changed my life and doing my research on both the medical and dental professions, the decision came easily. I was going to be a dentist.

Both Lyndsay and I attended dental school on an Army Health Services scholarship; the army paid our tuition and gave us a stipend for books and lab equipment. We spent thirteen weeks at an officer training course, and after graduating from four years of dental school, we did one year of general dentistry at Fort Gordon in Augusta, Georgia, before our residency, where we were technically on active duty. There was little chance of being deployed, however, and I was able to focus on dentistry. Since Fort Gordon is such a huge base, I had a vast number of patients. You name it; I saw it and got to treat it while we were there. After our three-year residencies, we were sent to Fort Drum in Upstate New York, where I was the chief of prosthodontics. Lyndsay and I were the cochairs of the Implant Board, where we developed treatment plans and provided implant therapy to the soldiers of the Tenth Mountain Division, which was stationed there.

When you graduate from dental school and pass your boards, you are licensed to practice anything under the scope of dentistry, but I wasn't interested in general dentistry. I didn't want to just do root canals or bone grafts for the rest of my life. Instead, the idea of being a prosthodontist intrigued me. I loved the problem solving involved in prosthodontics, being able to jump in on a complicated case and come up with solutions. I was fascinated by the technology and advancements in dental prosthetics and felt energized by the thought of working on complex dental issues. I decided to specialize, and so I spent three years in a prosthodontic residency focusing solely on restoring and replacing missing or broken teeth. I didn't do any root canals. I didn't perform any surgeries. I didn't do anything but prosthodontics.

During my prosthodontic residency, I worked long days—often sixty or seventy hours a week—and because the residents in all the specialties were housed together in one building, I was able to easily collaborate with my colleagues and learn from them. There was a lot of interaction across teams. I learned not only the prosthodontic aspect of treatment but also how all the different parts of the mouth interacted by following the treatment of patients from the initial consultation right up until the finish. This knowledge has helped me immeasurably in my ability to construct comprehensive treatment plans for all my patients.

My patients are extremely important to me, and I treat them with the same love and compassion with which I treat my own family members. Dentistry is very much a family affair, since my wife is a periodontist. We are self-confessed dental geeks, and we like nothing better than talking about our patients or the newest, greatest thing to come down the dental technology pipeline, even across the dinner table or during long car rides with our three children. Lyndsay and I like to joke that they're our mini dental apprentices. They're especially intrigued by the personal stories of our patients' treatments and love following the progress. It's rewarding to see the excitement on their faces when we tell them that we've finally fitted the crowns for this patient or that we were able to successfully treat that patient. Of course, they are occasionally bored silly when we get into the nuts and bolts of it, and then they simply roll their eyes and indulge us. They're great and caring kids and have been brought up knowing there is no shame in having dental damage; there is only compassion and solutions.

In my experience, people will avoid seeing a dentist for three reasons, and the most common is shame. They fear they'll be viewed as lazy or stupid for not dealing with their dental issues, and they frequently feel guilty for letting things get to a desperate point. Often, they are afraid they're going to shock me. Many people are convinced that when I look into their mouths, I'm going to see the worst things I've ever encountered. Believe me, that's pretty unlikely. The majority of the time, it's really no big deal, and we can put a plan in place and get them all fixed up. My team works hard to put patients at ease and remove any trace of shame they might feel. What's happened with their teeth is in the past; we're not here to shame or judge them. We're here to make them feel comfortable and excited about their treatment.

I also meet quite a few patients who have avoided dental treatment out of fear. There's a whole generation of folks out there who've had terrible experiences with dental care in their lives, often because they endured pain due to a dentist avoiding the use of an anesthetic, either because they didn't want to use it or it wasn't available. Treating a patient without numbing them—especially an anxious patient—can rarely be justified. It turns a dental visit into a nightmare and creates negative associations in a patient's mind. Most of the practices I know bend over backward to make a visit to the dentist a positive experience. At my practice, we take the time to work with these patients before beginning treatment to reassure them the experience is going to be far less intense or painful than they anticipated. Dentistry has become much more patient friendly and focused on the feelings the patient has about treatment. Our core value at my dental practice is to focus on the patient's experience. We want them to be comfortable and relaxed and to actually enjoy coming to see us. We love our patients, and it means the world to us to have them experience a nice warm environment and feel comfortable with the care we give them.

The third common reason people avoid going to the dentist is financial. Let's face it, dental care can be expensive, especially care that involves multiple implants, surgery, or full mouth reconstruction. People rationalize their avoidance of dental care by convincing themselves that tooth issues are no big deal. What many don't realize is that oral health is, in fact, a huge deal, and ignoring it can cause damage in other parts of the body. We understand that not everyone

Oral health is, in fact, a huge deal, and ignoring it can cause damage in other parts of the body.

can afford the dental care they need, so a regular part of our practice is assisting patients with the financial aspect of care. The majority of my patients are in the middle to upper range of the socioeconomic scale, with a few at the lower end. We work with a handful of really helpful financial institutions that provide zero-interest or low-interest loans that folks can pay back over a longer period of time. Many times, we can help patients avoid a large up-front cost and instead figure out ways to budget the expense so it becomes manageable. We'll do as much as we can to get patients into our office and get them fixed up.

It is extremely important to me that a patient has complete faith and confidence in my ability to help them. Your dental care is always your choice. It's your mouth. If you're not simpatico with your dentist or if your personalities just don't click, there's nothing wrong with finding someone else to help you.

As you might have guessed by now, I really am passionate about dentistry and my patients. That's why I've written this book. I hope to educate, reassure, and encourage people who have questions, fears, or doubts. I want to show just how much better we can make your life with dentistry.

I want to share my excitement at the great technological advances that have been made in the field of prosthodontics. Cases that seemed impossible to solve years ago are now seen daily and are successfully treated with little or no pain. This is not your grandma's dental care. Offices are warm and inviting, staff is sympathetic and understanding, and technology is state of the art. No one should live with mouth pain, missing or broken teeth, and embarrassment.

In my practice, I aim both to fix difficult problems and to teach patients how to care for themselves once they leave the office. I believe in guiding my patients on a disciplined path of oral care and regular checkups. Remember, an ounce of prevention is worth a pound of cure, as hokey as that may sound. If we can catch problems early, we can prevent a world of difficulty that will inevitably happen. Above all, I want to reassure patients that they have options and that I am 100 percent certain I can help. There is just no such thing as a hopeless case.

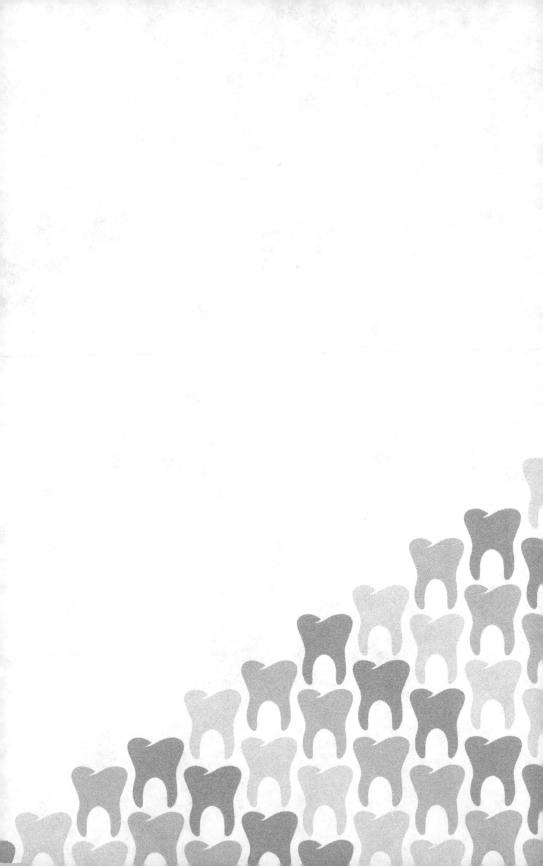

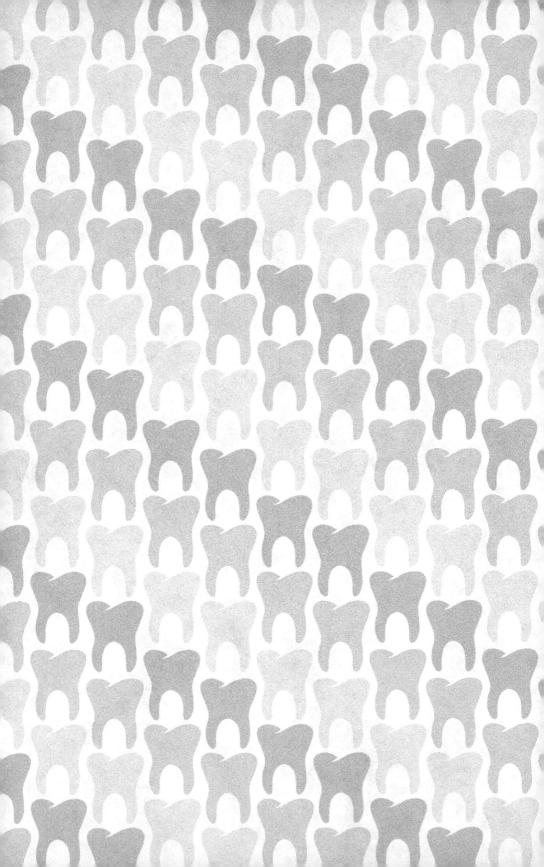

CHAPTER 1

"What Is a Prosthodontist, and Why Should I See One?"

uring my prosthodontic residency, I met a young warrant officer—he was probably in his early thirties—who came to me with his mouth in terrible shape and his spirits deflated. He had neglected his dental health for so long that the last dentist he saw told him his only option was to get a full set of dentures. I really didn't want that to happen, especially for such a young guy. I immediately had him examined by an oral surgeon and a periodontist, and then, after my own examination, I put together a treatment plan that included extensive work from a number of specialists.

And guess what? We were able to save the majority of his natural teeth and restore most of the missing ones. When all was said and done, he had a mouth full of twenty-eight beautiful, functional teeth. The difference from the start to the conclusion of treatment was dazzling. Here was a young, single man who was torn up by the fact that he'd have to wear dentures for the rest of his life, worried about what would happen if he lost his dentures while deployed and fearful that if he flirted with a girl, they might slip out and embarrass him.

He was aware of the challenges that come with dentures and wanted us to save as many of his teeth as possible, which is what we did. The results were both esthetically and functionally awesome, and this young guy, who used to cover his mouth with his hand when he smiled, had the biggest grin on his face when he walked out of the office. His new smile gave him tremendous confidence. For me, the rewards of giving him a healthy and functional mouth were nearly equal to the rewards of seeing his self-esteem skyrocket and watching him leave with a spring in his step that had been missing before. I think this was the first time I saw how skilled dental care can truly change someone's life. Each case like this inspires me to learn more and do more for my patients.

I hear you wondering "What exactly is prosthodontics?" and I could simply tell you it's an awesome, fascinating, technologically advanced dental specialty that uses state-of-the-art equipment and materials, but it's even more than that. Prosthodontics is one of about a dozen dental specialties—you've heard of some, like oral surgery, orthodontics, and periodontics—and is defined by the American Dental Association as "a dental specialty pertaining to the diagnosis, treatment planning, rehabilitation, and maintenance of the oral function, comfort, appearance, and health of patients with clinical conditions associated with missing or deficient teeth and/or oral and maxillofacial tissues using biocompatible substitutes."

That's quite a mouthful, I know, but it's quite a specialty, and that's why I love it! During my residency, I trained in both removable prosthodontics (dentures, partials) and fixed prosthodontics (crowns, bridges, implants), and I use both in my practice.

It was during my residency that I realized the unique value of prosthodontics and became aware of the importance of being part of a skilled team handling cases. A complex case would often involve an oral surgeon, an endodontist, and a periodontist, for example. Everybody would look to the prosthodontist to assimilate all the information and come up with a plan. I like to think of the prosthodontist as the quarterback of treatment. We see the whole picture of the field and then coordinate getting the patient to all the other specialists, let them do their areas of the treatment plan to perfection, and put it all together at the end. It's a real team effort, and everyone has to do their part.

If teeth need to be removed or a root canal is indicated or implants need to be placed, we use a coordinated timeline and make sure everything in the mouth is supported through the whole task. Then, once all the pieces are in place, I will come in and do the final crowns, buildups, or dental prosthesis—whatever we planned for. The treatment plan is vital, and when everyone does their part in the right sequence with the right plan, everything goes smoothly. I

Don't listen if someone tells you that you are a hopeless case, because you absolutely are not.

carefully plan for all my cases, whether they call for a simple implant or a full mouth reconstruction.

Considering the success of that first full mouth reconstruction on the young officer, I am saddened when I think of people who give up hope of finding a solution that works for them. I promise you there is always something we can do to help, whether it's crowns, implants, partial dentures, or even full dentures. Don't listen if someone tells you that you are a hopeless case, because you absolutely are not.

Maybe you've just seen the wrong dentist! Dentists are people, too, and sometimes a patient and a dentist might not be the right fit. One dentist may be really good at what he does, though he might have trouble with apprehensive patients. Another may be great at putting patients at ease, but they haven't been trained to use the latest technology. Whatever the reason, it's important that you find a dentist you feel completely comfortable with and confident in who is familiar with the recent incredible advancements in dentistry.

Once you've found a dentist you are comfortable with, the sky's the limit when it comes to your treatment options. Okay, maybe not the sky, but certainly the ceiling of a large indoor stadium. You get the picture. There are a ton of choices: implants, crowns, partials—we do them all. Even those treatments that you've seen in commercials that advertise "teeth in a day" or "a smile in a day." Really! Technology has advanced to the point that now, if a patient has a mouth full of unhealthy teeth—to the point where we can't restore or save them or if their bite is so far off because of the damage—we have the ability to fix them up in a most remarkable way.

As with any procedure, we start first with a treatment plan, then lay out the groundwork and determine everything we need, usually also working with an oral surgeon and a periodontist. Once this is done, the patient can come in for surgery, where the surgeon removes the unhealthy teeth and we put in five or six implants. During that same appointment, I can also attach a realistic set of teeth and gums to those implants, and the patient can go home that day with everything in place—a smile in a day.

These kinds of procedures are awesome, but of course it's not like saying, "Abracadabra!" and boom, you're all set. A great deal of work goes into the planning alone, and you've got to have a great surgeon. I'm blessed to work with some gifted surgeons. We plan it all out and do the work, and patients leave with a temporary appliance that looks like a whole set of teeth. In about six months they come back, and I can install the permanent ones. So, they walk in with a mouth full of terrible teeth and leave with a full set of really nice-looking teeth. It's a pretty awesome thing we can do in one day.

The ability to use the latest technology and treat even the most difficult cases is a direct result of the intensive training involved in becoming a specialist. A prosthodontist puts in eleven years of education after high school. I like to joke with my kids that when my wife, Lyndsay—who is a periodontist—and I finally graduated from our residencies, we were graduating from the twenty-third grade. There's a lot of training involved! The most valuable thing I got out of my training and residency was the exposure to a vast amount of information and a wide variety of complicated cases. It helps me to be very open-minded when it comes to treatment options and to remember that not every patient gets the same treatment planning. There are so many variables that must be factored in that a "one size fits all" plan is impossible.

My exposure during my residency to different dental specialists and treatment modalities definitely influenced my process and approach to cases. It was a very collaborative effort, and I learned an enormous amount, which prepared me to deal with just about any dental situation that comes through my door.

One interesting thing I discovered over the course of my training—and something I still see to this day—is that it's pretty common for people to be missing teeth through no fault of their own. Sometimes teeth just aren't there in the first place. (This is called hypodontia, a developmental absence of one or more teeth.)

Sometimes this missing tooth might cause an aesthetic problem if it's near the front of the mouth, and since it's never a good idea to ignore missing teeth, this would be something to call a prosthodontist about. Sometimes it's possible to close the gap using orthodontics, and people should know that even if you have a healthy mouth, it's important to replace teeth that, for whatever reason, just failed to come in.

Occasionally, I am called to rescue a patient from a situation where they received treatment without a comprehensive plan in place. I've seen cases where a patient has a complicated bite or worn-down teeth, and a simple plan just didn't solve the problem.

Let's say the bottom teeth are a little worn down and the top front teeth are pretty small. Someone might just put in crowns to make them bigger, thinking the mouth will be okay with the new teeth. But this can cause a lot of trouble, since the back teeth need to provide adequate support for the front teeth. Things can get complicated quickly, and you need someone who can plan for those complications. The mouth is a very harmonious environment, and all the pieces have to work together. Teeth aren't just for looks or for chewing; it doesn't work that way. They've all got to function together.

Another issue I see frequently is the threat of tooth loss because of periodontal disease—bone loss and gum loss—and I've been referred to by periodontists to treat this situation. Periodontal disease causes people to lose teeth they didn't think they would lose because, although they don't have decay or cavities, when they start to lose that bone and tissue, all of a sudden there's less and less tooth anchored in the bone. A prosthodontist can create a plan of action, get ahead of the bone loss, and get working on a solution.

One of my most memorable cases involved an US Air Force fighter pilot I treated at Fort Drum. His stressful job caused him to grind his teeth so ferociously that he was wearing them down at an alarming pace. At the rate he was going, he would have no teeth left in a few years. Fortunately, after receiving clearance from my commanding officer to clear my schedule to focus on one patient, we were able to do a full mouth reconstruction within one week. We gave him crowns, then fixed and protected all of his remaining teeth. He went from a mouth full of worn-down and damaged teeth to a mouth full of beautiful, healthy teeth—all in a week's time! This case really stuck with me because it was early on in my career, and it was one of the more dramatic improvements I've ever seen. With the help of an amazing lab technician who worked tirelessly to create the permanent crowns, we completed twenty-eight crowns in only five days—an operation that is usually completed in stages over the course of a year.

There are endless situations that cause people to lose teeth, and many times it's through no fault of their own. I had a patient whose chemotherapy treatments caused him to lose all but two of his teeth. The remaining teeth were tiny little stumps and not in very good condition, so I was unable to make an impression. We ended up doing a digital scan of his top teeth and his bottom jaw and sent that to a lab, and they 3D printed a denture for his bottom teeth. About two weeks later, we were able to custom fit the denture around his remaining two teeth. He went from dealing with a desperate situation to having a nice, stable prosthesis so he could chew and function.

Didn't I tell you? We'll always find a solution!

There is no such thing as a hopeless case. Of course, the best thing is to hang on to what God gave you, but that isn't always possible. With removable appliances like dentures, patients regain only about 30 percent of their chewing ability. (Yes, they've actually done experiments involving people chewing peanuts and spitting, but I won't torture you with the details.) Implants give a patient about 75 to 80 percent of their chewing ability back, and that's certainly an acceptable ratio. Even in the worst cases, we can figure out a fix. My team and I have extensive experience and have seen just about everything, so if you're thinking you have something going on in your mouth that I've never seen before, think again. The possibility of that is minimal.

For me, being a dentist is a dream come true. I've always been drawn to the helping professions and to problem solving, so it's been a perfect fit. When I'm presented with a complicated case, I love that I have both the knowledge and the resources to put together a plan of treatment. Using all the things I learned in dental school, my residency, and my practice allows me to tell even the most desperate patient, "Hey, I can help you" and have the confidence to know I can.

Now that you know there are many options for dealing with missing and broken teeth, I'd like to tell you a little secret. People with a mouth full of straight, white teeth are not necessarily in possession of great oral health. Lurking under that splendid smile could be a world of trouble just waiting to show itself. There's much more to oral health than shiny white teeth, and it's important to know what you're up against when it comes to the many and varied ways your oral health can be compromised.

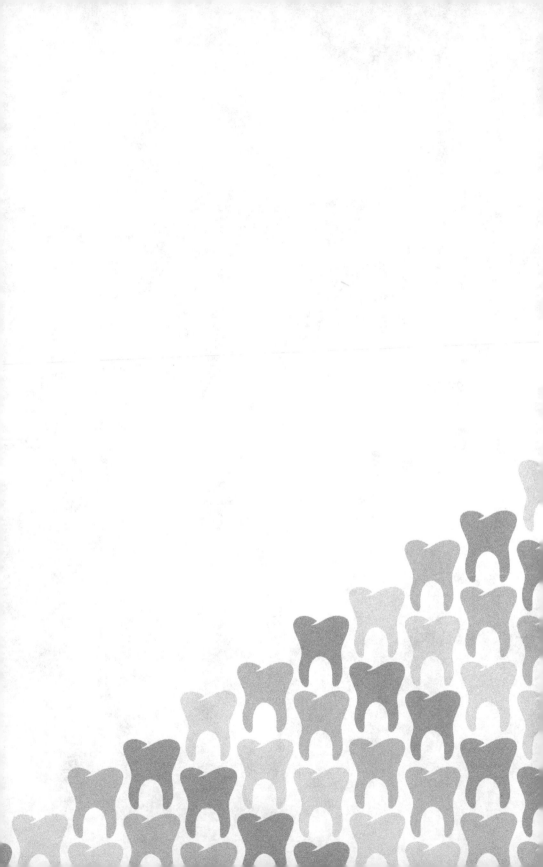

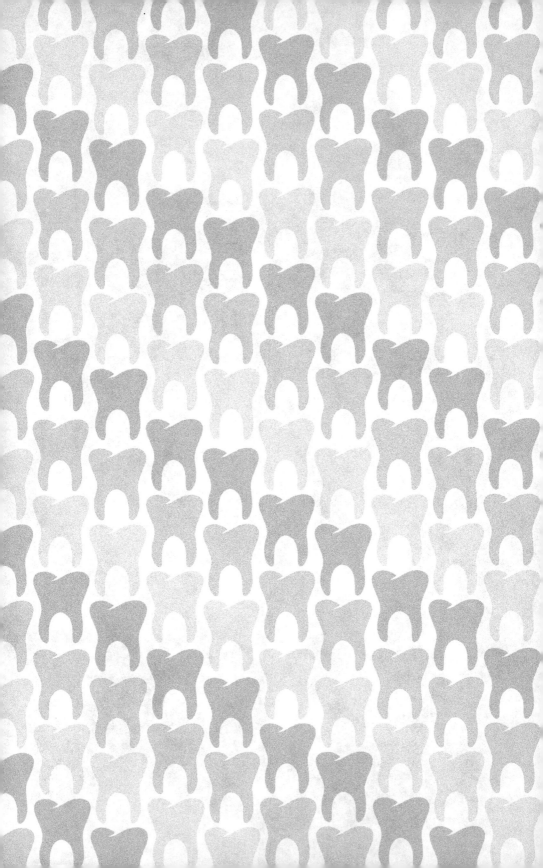

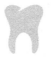

"My Teeth Are Straight and White, So They're Good"

Y ou've just finished your morning routine and can't resist smiling at yourself in the mirror, admiring your straight and dazzling white teeth. You might even imagine you see a little sparkle like in those old toothpaste commercials. You say to yourself, "I've got this! My teeth are in prime condition." But are they?

Well, maybe not. It might be a mistake to prematurely congratulate yourself on your brilliant dental health. A number of conditions and diseases exist for which there are no symptoms and that can't be detected by the naked eye. Periodontal disease, for example—an infection of the tissues and bone that hold your teeth in place—can sneak up and attack with subtle symptoms or even no symptoms. In some ways it's similar to heart disease. You might look and feel fine, not noticing much going on, but you could have underlying disease.

In my practice, I see people in their thirties and forties who have undiagnosed periodontal disease that has reached the point where it threatens their teeth. Some of these issues can only be detected using radiographs and bone-level measurements, just like some heart disease can only be detected by specific tests. You could also have erosion and breakdown of the tooth enamel, which you might not be able to detect just yet. "But I take care of myself, and I eat healthy foods," you may say. "How could this happen?"

Believe it or not, periodontal disease and eroding teeth can be caused by some of the very things you are doing that you think are beneficial for your health.

We're all encouraged to drink plenty of water to stay healthy, and if we work out strenuously, we're told to replace our electrolytes by drinking products like Gatorade. The problem is that some of these drinks—yes, even some bottled waters—have insane pH levels that act like battery acid on your teeth. The pH figure reveals how acidic or alkaline something is. A neutral pH is 7, and the normal pH level in a person's mouth is around 6. The lower the pH, the higher the acidity, and when the teeth are exposed to lower pH levels, the minerals in your teeth become very unhappy. Most people are aware that sugary drinks like Coke and sweet tea are not the best for their health, but in my experience, many folks are unaware that the low pH levels in soda can wreak havoc on teeth. When you consider the low pH, the high sugar content, and the carbonation in soda, you may be looking at public enemy number one in the dental world. To put it in context, water has a neutral pH of 7. Classic Coke has a pH of 2.4 and 10 teaspoons of sugar. Dr. Pepper's pH is 2.9 and also has 10 teaspoons of sugar. And then there's the problem with bottled water.

It's hard for most people to imagine getting through the day without consuming at least some bottled water. It's so convenient!

You can purchase it just about anywhere, and by carrying it with you, you won't have to rely on unsanitary public water fountains or water of unknown origins coming out of faucets.

However, bottled water can actually pose a threat to your teeth.

I hear you thinking "Say it ain't so!" but unfortunately it's the truth. Bottled water can be super acidic and can throw off the pH levels in the mouth to the point where the enamel begins to erode. This is not a good thing. Your mouth wants to stay at a pH level of around 6, and bathing your teeth in low-pH bottled water all day doesn't allow that to happen. This constant acidic climate will begin to cause damage, and sometimes you won't even know it's happening. You think you're doing the right thing by drinking plenty of water, but it's really important to be careful and check the pH levels of the bottled water you consume, or you'll be setting yourself up for decay and tooth breakdown.

ACIDIC RANGE		NEUTRAL RANGE		ALKALINE RANGE	
4pH	5pH	6pH	7pH	8pH	9pH	10pH
Sports Drinks	Dasani	Poland Spring	Evian	Real Water	TEN Water
Soda	Aquafina	Crystal Geyser	FIJI	Icelandic	Aquahydrate
	Deer Park	Smartwater	Eternal	Evamor	Essentia
	Penta	Zephyrhills	Core	Alkaline 88	
		Tap Water	Lifewtr		
			Tap Water		

Source: "Is Your Bottled Water Acidic or Alkaline?" TenSpringWater.com, accessed December 16, 2022, https://www.tenspringwater.com/is-your-bottled-water-acidic-neutral-or-alkaline.

In addition to the damaging pH levels, bottled water doesn't contain fluoride, so your teeth miss out on one of the most beneficial things you can do to maintain good oral health. According to the Centers for Disease Control and Prevention, the fluoridation of water is one of the ten great public health achievements of the twentieth century.[1] I have seen the evidence of this in my practice.

When a new patient sits down in my chair and I have a look at their teeth, I can often tell whether they grew up in an area that had fluoridated water or well water. People who grow up without fluoridation in their water have what is often referred to as "soft" teeth, which puts them at greater risk of problems. As far as preventing decay and breakdown, fluoridated water is right up there with aggressive preventative care and advancements in home oral care tools like the Waterpik. People used to lose their teeth at a much earlier age, but with these advancements, they're keeping them far longer. I recently treated a patient who still had the majority of her teeth at age ninety-

Fluoride is essential in protecting our teeth.

eight! Sure, she had a lot of fillings and crowns, but I'm pretty sure that part of the reason she's kept those teeth so long has to do with fluoride.

Fluoride is essential in protecting our teeth , and the amount of money people have saved on dental work because of fluoridation is staggering. But even fluoride can't protect your teeth from everything. People are living much longer than they did years ago, and our diets have changed dramatically. We've introduced sugar into nearly every meal we eat, and we consume fewer of the foods that are tooth friendly. It's best to stick to less-damaging snacks like apples, pears, or cheese. It's our job to combat the enemies that threaten our oral health.

---

1   Center for Disease Control, "Ten Great Public Health Achievements—United States, 1900–1999," accessed December 16, 2022, https://www.cdc.gov/mmwr/preview/mmwrhtml/00056796.htm.

So, now you're thinking that I've spoiled drinks like Coke and sweet tea for you, haven't I? Don't worry! There's a solution, and it's all about the *way* you consume these drinks. You can counteract the damaging effects of the ingredients in your favorite beverages by just drinking smarter. Basically, if you are a sipper and love nothing more than keeping a can of Coke or a glass of sweet tea on your desk, taking sip after sip all day long, that's going to cause a lot more trouble than if you just drink it down in one fell swoop. The sipping bathes your teeth in an acidic and sugary environment all day and does tons of damage.

When I was in the army, I treated countless soldiers who would drink Red Bull or Monster all day or all night long, and boy, that stuff is just toxic to teeth. It was like a continuous bath of acid on the teeth for hours and hours on end.

My advice is to drink your soda or sweet tea in one sitting, maybe with your lunch, and then rinse your mouth out with water a few times. Just swishing some water around in your mouth after enjoying a sweet drink will knock out 90-plus percent of the residual sugars.

Sugary drinks and low pH water aren't the only enemies of your teeth. I see all kinds of damage done by a wide range of things people eat, and some might surprise you. I have seen a lot of trouble caused by people sucking on cough drops, for example. They'll pop one in their mouth, and it will sit all cozied up to a tooth as it dissolves, creating a treacherous environment. I notice this a lot with my older patients; they seem to love cough drops. This same situation can happen with anything that's full of sugar and meant to be dissolved slowly in your mouth. It sits there doing its devilish work, and you end up with decay, causing cavities and even destroying the area surrounding fillings. The tooth can start to erode around the filling, and all of a sudden the filling doesn't have a strong enough bond and starts to loosen—and that's trouble.

One of the most astonishingly damaging things I've seen for teeth has to be frozen Milk Duds. I had a patient whose favorite treat was these little frozen demons. I'm sure they're delicious, but they are a perfect storm of dental danger: sugar, caramel, and freezing cold. Another popular culprit is the frozen Snickers bar, since it adds rock-hard nuts to the recipe for disaster.

Before you vow to give up all sugary treats, it's important to remember that hazards to your teeth come in many disguises, and not all of them contain sugar. In fact, for me, the number one culprit of all dental damage has to be popcorn. I see a lot of patients who have broken teeth on unpopped kernels. There they are, happily and healthily snacking away, and *bam!* It's like biting down on a pebble, and it can cause a terrible fracture of the tooth.

But it's not only the unpopped kernels that cause issues; it's also those annoying little husks. The husk of a piece of popcorn is shaped very similarly to the curve of a tooth. Those hard little husks slide right down in between your tooth and gum tissue and just won't budge. It's like they're custom fit to your tooth! I've seen people come in after attacking the problem with a toothpick, causing all kinds of damage to the gum. I've also seen a husk work its way down into the area between the tooth and gum, and no amount of poking or prodding will get it out.

The only solution is to make a small incision in the gum to extract the husk. It sounds unbelievable, but it's more common than you could imagine. So, even though popcorn is a healthy snack, it's probably best to avoid it, or at the very least, check carefully for unpopped kernels. If you get a husk stuck on a tooth, try some floss rather than a toothpick; you could save yourself some painful gums and avoid a dentist visit. If you do get a stubborn husk caught between your teeth, it's worth a quick trip to the dentist for some assistance, and we promise we won't chuckle. We really have treated this before!

Popcorn is certainly not the only healthy snack that can cause damage. Ice cubes, hard nuts, Pennsylvania Dutch pretzels (you know the ones—they're hard as a rock), and frozen grapes are all up there when it comes to foods that can damage your teeth. Chewing these snacks takes a lot of grinding power and can be particularly hazardous to older patients or those with compromised teeth. To make things worse, frozen snacks can cause the teeth to become brittle, adding to the equation. Although tooth enamel is the hardest substance in the human body, it's no match for ice. Ice can crack or chip teeth, damage dental appliances like braces, and dislodge fillings. So, the next time you find yourself casually chewing away on ice cubes, please just stop.

Now that I've burst your snacking bubble, I'd like to get back to your dazzling smile—the one you admired in the mirror this morning. Sure, it looks marvelous, and those front top and bottom six teeth ("the Social Six") are stunning, but my concern is what lurks beyond. I've had patients whose "smiling teeth" are fine, but when I take a closer look, I often find back teeth bombed out and broken down. People tend not to worry about these teeth because nobody sees them, and while there's a certain logic to that, the fact is that back teeth have a job to do, and if they're missing or in poor condition, you may be using your front teeth to do work they weren't intended to do. The front teeth are designed to cut food and then send it to the back for the big guys to do all the grinding and chewing. When you don't have healthy back teeth to do this work, you use your front teeth, which were not designed to grind and chew. Those teeth will begin to break down a lot faster than they should, and that's not a good thing. If you don't have back teeth working efficiently, the forces and pressures put on your front teeth are enormous and quite damaging.

Every so often I have patients come in and tell me their front teeth are starting to look a little worse for wear and want to get some crowns to spruce things up. When I examine them, I see that the teeth in the back are not able to support the ones in front, causing the front teeth to wear down. That could turn into a full mouth reconstruction where I have to reestablish the bite in the back. The patient comes in thinking it's a small deal, and sometimes it turns out to be just the opposite.

Occasionally a patient may come in for a checkup and be taken by surprise when I discover some serious issues going on in teeth that neither look too bad nor cause any pain or sensitivity. For whatever reason, sometimes the nerve doesn't become triggered, perhaps because it starts to pull back or regress a little bit. If the nerve pulls back at the same rate as the decay, it creates a kind of buffer, and the patient may feel little or no discomfort. Many times I find what I call "balloon" cavities, where there's a tiny hole or black spot on the chewing surface, and the patient thinks it's a little stain or the start of a small cavity. But when I look at this on an X-ray, I see that this tiny little spot has just ballooned underneath the surface and taken out a ton of healthy tooth. So, what looks like no big deal to the naked eye can be a situation that requires a root canal, a crown, or even an extraction. Another good reason to go for regular checkups: catch and prevent. Catch and *prevent*. I can't say it enough. My mission is to prevent people from having massive discomfort caused by something that could have been treated if caught at an earlier stage.

Preventative care is vitally important for oral health, but hanging on to your teeth isn't the only reason you want to see a dentist regularly. What's going on in your mouth can affect your entire body. Take, for example, patients who come to me with a mouth full of broken and decayed teeth. They are in pain—sometimes terrible pain. They literally can't function. Within two weeks of taking out all the teeth and clearing the infection, they start to see systemic changes in their bodies. Their sleeping improves; their attitude is more positive. In all the years I've been practicing, I've never seen anyone who wasn't extremely happy to have broken, bombed-out teeth gone.

The impact oral decay and infection have on the body and mind can't be understated, since they can affect everything from the cardiovascular system to the nervous system. Abscesses, unchecked decay, periodontal disease, and bone loss are all related to infection. And this infection doesn't just stay in your mouth. There is a 100 percent correlation to infection and inflammation in the mouth and cardiovascular inflammation. Dentists working with medical professionals have discovered that the exact same plaque bacteria in your mouth can be found lining the arteries of the heart. Inflammation of the cardiovascular system is a huge indicator of upcoming problems like strokes. And, in extreme cases, you can have an infection in the mouth that travels to the sinus cavities or brain and has the potential to cause death. The good news is that if you have a nice, healthy, clean mouth, you don't have inflammation or plaque that will find its way to your arteries.

I don't want to scare you silly; fatalities are an extreme situation. But it can happen. Again, that's why it's always best to get yourself in for regular checkups, pain or no pain. A toothache is nature's way of telling you there's a problem brewing, but why let it get to that point?

I hope I've taught you a few things and convinced you that even if your teeth look straight and white and you're not experiencing any discomfort, there may be trouble brewing behind that perfect smile. Here's what I'd like you to keep in mind as you go about your routine:

1. Watch what you eat and drink. Even healthy foods can be hazardous to your dental health, so try to avoid anything that's sticky, sweet, and hard. It's best to stay away from frozen Milk Duds (and frozen Snickers, frozen Milky Ways, etc.), ice cubes, and popcorn. If life is just not worth living without your daily dose of sweet tea or soda, at least drink wisely. No day-long sipping. Be aware of the pH levels in the bottled water you choose, and make sure you get your fluoride (think "fluoridated" toothpaste).

2. Don't be fooled into believing that your "smiling teeth" are an indication of what's going on in the dark recesses of your mouth. It's best to have a dentist check you out to make sure everything's in good order.

3. Oral health affects every aspect of your body, from your cardiovascular system to your nervous system. Your goal is to have a healthy, clean mouth, free from infection and inflammation.

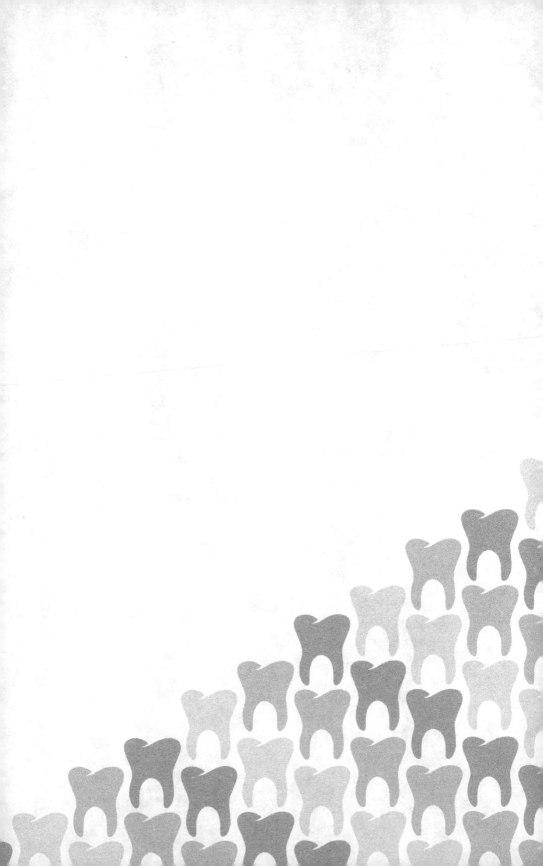

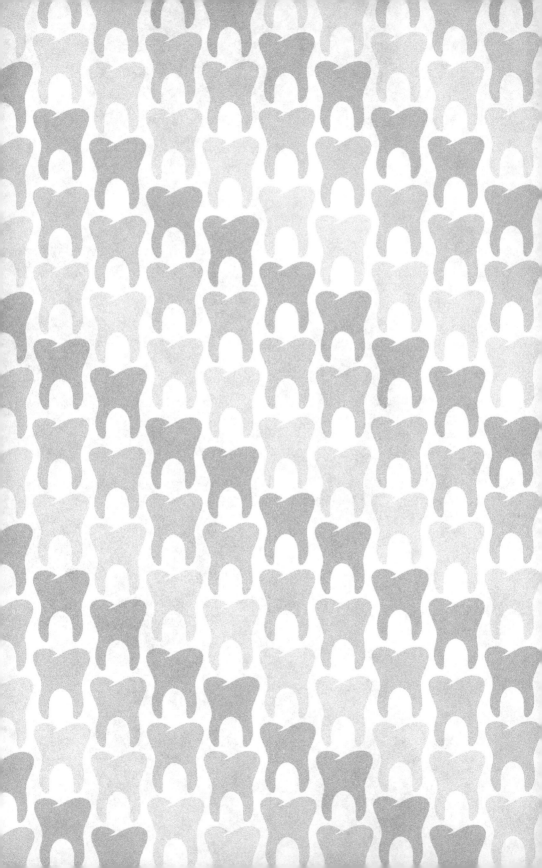

"I'm Only Missing One Tooth—What's the Big Deal?"

You're missing a tooth and telling yourself, "I have so many other teeth. What's missing one tooth if other people can't even see that it's missing?"

Well, I'm here to tell you that even one single missing tooth can cause trouble. When you lose a tooth, the majority of the time the rest of your teeth are going to start shifting, and all of a sudden you're putting different forces and different pressure on the wrong teeth. Although shifting teeth is relatively painless, the longer you wait, the more complicated and involved it becomes to restore or replace that missing space.

> **Even one single missing tooth can cause trouble.**

Our teeth were designed in a very specific way, and they work together as a team. So, over time, you'll come to find that the teeth next to the gap will start to lean in, and before you know it, you're not chewing on a full tooth surface; you're chewing on a corner or the edge of a tooth. It's just a matter of time before one or both of the surrounding teeth will be negatively affected. They could break or get beaten down, and then your problem is compounded. It's really best to tend to a missing tooth as soon as possible to avoid additional damage. Luckily, there are four different options to replace the missing tooth and get everything back in order.

The first option is to do nothing, and honestly, that's rarely the right solution. But if it's the very last tooth in the back of your mouth and it doesn't have a chewing partner, most likely nothing else is going to move, so doing nothing can be the solution. Sometimes we'll have patients who need to have the very back tooth taken out, but since they weren't using it for chewing anyway, I'll tell them it's not worth the time and investment to replace it. They're not going to miss it. The combined chewing function of the second molars is only about 5 percent anyway, so there really is no need to replace those.

The next option would be to make something removable, like a partial denture. Partial dentures with a metal frame are the most common. The metal frame becomes a sturdy support for chewing, particularly if you're missing molars. These partial dentures are not permanent; you take them in and out. So, you wake up in the morning, pop it in, and it looks and acts like a natural tooth. You can chew and talk, and at the end of the day, you take it out so the gum tissue can heal overnight. It seems like overkill to deal with just one missing tooth, but it's the least expensive option, and that's what people will sometimes choose.

I have to point out that this solution requires a properly constructed replacement. If the replacement tooth is poorly constructed and installed without the right planning, it can put undue forces on the adjacent teeth and cause problems. When it's designed correctly and has the proper encompassing support, it'll be just fine. Some people opt for acrylic partials because of the lower cost, but I don't recommend them as a long-term solution, since they don't last. The majority of the time I use a state-of-the-art flexible acrylic or a nylon partial because I think they're far superior. Partials made from these materials are more esthetic because the metal doesn't show. They're more comfortable because as the thermoplastic material sits in your warm mouth all day, it molds and shapes to your actual gum tissue, making it more comfortable and more snug. It doesn't put a lot of torque or pressure on the remaining teeth, so you don't have to worry about damaging your other teeth.

Option number three would be installing bridgework, which entails preparing the teeth on either side of the gap for crowns and making a three-piece unit that gets cemented over the top. Crowns that are made of high-tech dental porcelains look just like natural teeth. This is a great option when the teeth on either side of the gap would benefit from a crown anyway because they have fillings, are unaesthetic, or aren't in the right location. We can kill two birds with one stone using this technique. We replace the missing tooth and correct the adjacent teeth all in the same procedure. The bridge is cemented in place and has an average lifespan of about ten years, but that's only the average. I see patients who had bridges installed in the 1970s that are still looking and working just fine.

The staying power of a bridge depends largely on the quality of the dentist, the condition of the patient's mouth, and the home care it is given. Bridges require a larger investment, but they're a great long-term solution to the problem of a missing tooth. We take great pains to match the shade of the patient's natural teeth, and bridges are nearly undetectable to the naked eye.

Our last option is to replace a missing tooth using a single-tooth implant. We put a titanium screw into the jawbone, and it fuses to the bone. We let that heal for a few months so that the screw fuses completely to the bone, and then we bring the patient back in and cement or attach a tooth-colored crown to it. This is a more expensive option, but for a lot of patients it's a great one because the implant functions in virtually the identical way a natural tooth does, and it's permanent. Implants are indistinguishable from natural teeth and allow you to chew, speak, and smile with confidence, since they won't slip or shift. Implants won't hurt surrounding teeth, and you'll never get a cavity in them. If they're cared for like your natural teeth, they'll last a lifetime, and they will also prevent bone loss in the jaw.

I'd like to say a few words about bone loss, since it is an important issue when it comes to missing teeth—even just one. Bone is living tissue that needs stimulation to stay healthy. A tooth anchored in your jaw gives the bone the stimulation it needs to survive. Without it, the bone will begin to disappear. While only one missing tooth probably won't cause terrible issues, the more teeth you're missing, the more at risk your jaw will be to fractures and injury. If a lot of teeth are missing, it can visibly change the appearance of your face, causing a sunken look. Implants offer the advantage of keeping the bone healthy, and they're a great option.

To summarize, my advice to you is not to underestimate the potential problems that can be caused by even one missing tooth. You have several options, and all of them are better than doing nothing (unless, as I said, it's one of those far back teeth). Dental technology is working in your favor by giving you choices that people didn't have years ago. Removable appliances, bridges, implants—you have lots of choices! By replacing that missing tooth, you'll be protecting the health of the surrounding teeth and the jawbone. And if that missing tooth is in a conspicuous place in your mouth, you'll feel better about yourself when you smile.

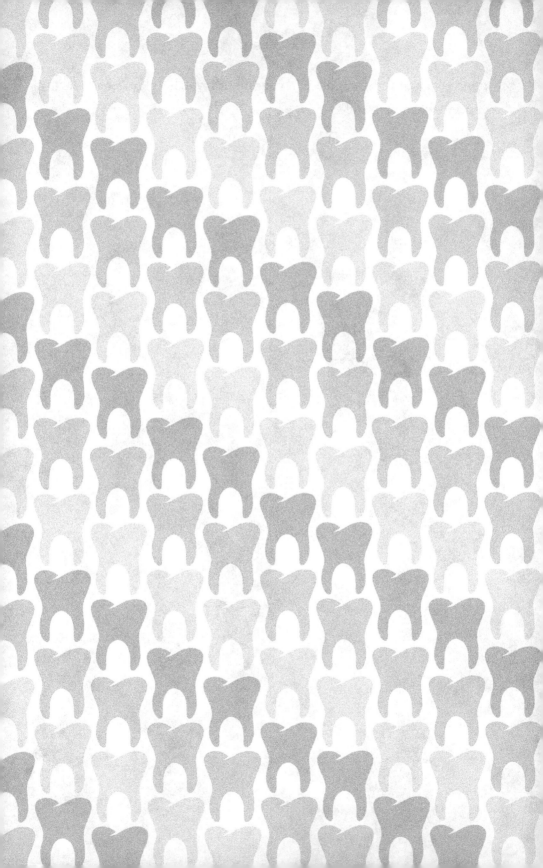

CHAPTER 4

"I've Lost Quite a Few Teeth—What Are My Options?"

For any number of reasons, you may find yourself in a situation where you've lost more than a few teeth and are wondering what your options are. Years ago, you would have had very few choices, but I'm happy to tell you that nowadays you have plenty. Everyone's situation is different, however, and having lots of options when it comes to replacing missing teeth will depend on your lifestyle, your budget, and a couple of other factors. *But*—we can only give you recommendations if you show up. There's no need to be ashamed of having missing teeth! Remember, we're here to help you, not to judge you. There are countless ways people lose teeth, and there is no point in assigning blame; our goal is to get you all fixed up—and believe me, it will change your life.

When I was at Fort Drum in upstate New York, the home of the Tenth Mountain Division and the most deployed unit in the army at the time, we had a great number of reservists who were called up. Many of these soldiers were coming from rural areas, and one of them, a young man from the backwoods of Louisiana, came to me in what can only be described as desperate shape. Although he was only in his early twenties, he had no teeth and wore a full set of very ill-fitting dentures. He was painfully embarrassed by his situation; he wouldn't smile, and he was terribly ashamed. He'd never even been on a date because of his situation. He told me a heartbreaking story of a time he was singing in his church choir and his denture fell out. As he told the story, I could feel the pain and shame he experienced. My heart went out to him, yet I was really excited because I knew I could help him and couldn't wait to get started.

After examining him and creating a treatment plan, we got to work. After a thorough exam, we put in the implant posts that would eventually hold the dentures and gave him a temporary set of teeth to use while the tissue healed and the bone fused to the posts. Once everything was healed, we gave him a full set of beautiful dentures that snapped onto the metal posts we'd implanted. They looked and functioned much like natural teeth, and for this young guy, it made all the difference in the world. His confidence went through the roof! Eventually he was deployed overseas, and when he went back home to Louisiana, he met a girl and got engaged!

This was the same hopeless and downtrodden guy who never dated, who hadn't kissed a girl, and whose entire social life centered on his missing teeth and ill-fitting dentures. His new smile gave him confidence in himself, lifted his spirits, and led to many wonderful experiences. If that isn't a life changer, then I don't know what is. I also want to stress that changing someone's life through dentistry isn't limited to replacing a whole mouth full of missing teeth. I've had patients who suffered terrible embarrassment and shame from a gap in their teeth or just crooked teeth. When you fix these issues, you give the person so much. It's the biggest, best makeover you can do, and it's powerful.

This soldier was in a situation where we had no choice but to give him a full denture because he had lost all his natural teeth. The snap-in dentures we used were a terrific option because the denture itself is supported by metal posts in the jaw. They give the patient a great chewing ability, and because they fit better, there is less friction on the gums. They're super comfortable and natural looking and have the added bonus of preserving the jawbone because of the metal implants.

In a situation where some natural teeth are still left, there are a few other options. The treatment will depend on the condition and number of remaining teeth and the general health of the mouth. My team and I begin with an assessment of general oral health and the condition of the teeth, gums, and jaw. There's no blanket approach, and of course we try to save as many natural teeth as we can. Sometimes saving the few remaining teeth is not the best course of action, and we might do a lot of work around teeth that end up failing in a few years anyway. If we determine it's not prudent to save at-risk teeth, we'll have the surgeon extract everything and basically start with a blank canvas. So, if you're down to just a few remaining teeth, chances are we're going to take them out and start fresh, because trying to mix and match doesn't always work so well.

After making the determination of which, if any, teeth we can save, I carefully work up a treatment plan, which may include tooth extractions, root canals, gum treatments, and/or bone grafting. Then we move on to choose between snap-in dentures, partial dentures, implants, or bridges. Some of these procedures are more involved than others, and the prices vary widely. My point is that there are a lot of options when you're missing a large number of teeth, and it's essential to work with your dentist to figure out what the best solution is for you. Ignoring the situation or thinking it's okay to go through life without teeth can have serious consequences for your oral health and your physical appearance. It's not just about your lack of a smile. When you lose teeth, you lose bone in your jaw. When that happens, it not only increases your risk of jaw fracture (as the bone becomes thinner); it causes the entire face to have a sunken appearance.

I hate to think of people living with shame or pain because they avoid the dentist. Incredibly, a surprising number of people who have access to free or affordable dental care don't use it! The biggest roadblocks to visiting the dentist that I've encountered are fear of pain, financial concern, and shame. I can assure you that all the nightmare stories you've heard about dental pain just don't apply anymore. We have all kinds of tricks up our sleeves to make you comfortable, and, if anything, we will relieve your pain, not cause it.

Sometimes people think that if they go to the dentist, they will be ridiculed or seen as a bad person because their teeth are in disrepair. This is not what happens, I promise. We are in the helping profession, and as I mentioned before—and will keep mentioning—we are not here to judge you. I promise, no matter how bad you think the situation in your mouth is, we've seen worse. We will do everything we can to reassure you and keep you from feeling bad. The only reason people don't seek dental care that I can understand is the financial aspect. Yes, dental care is expensive, and dental insurance has become all but useless. Some financial institutions that give low-interest or zero-interest loans for dental care do exist, but the reality is that many of the procedures cost a lot of money, and that's another reason I believe so strongly in prevention.

Even patients with the best oral care habits can find themselves in a situation where they need to have multiple teeth—or all their teeth—replaced. Because of the enormous strides that have been made in dental technology, we are able to do things we could never have done just a few years ago, and we're able to do them a lot faster and more efficiently. Once we have a proper treatment plan in place, we are now able to bring a patient who needs all their teeth removed into the office, sedate them if they so choose, remove the teeth, put in the implants, and attach new teeth to an implant—all in one day.

Conventionally, when we place an implant, we want to give it time for the new bone to grow onto the outside structure of the post. The most successful way to do a single implant is to place the implant, cover it over with tissue, and then let the bone heal over the course of a few months. We know that if you put a tooth on an implant right away, you run the risk of a patient putting too much pressure on it and thereby not allowing the bone

> **We are able to do things we could never have done just a few years ago, and we're able to do them a lot faster and more efficiently.**

and implant to fuse efficiently. Lately we are pushing the protocols to enable people to get replacement teeth much sooner. We can put on temporary crowns that are a bit smaller so people don't use the surface to bite with. We also warn folks not to overload the teeth, and when we do the multiple implants, we find that they don't get overloaded if the patient remembers not to put a lot of pressure on them. These practices can make a huge difference for people whose lives would be negatively impacted if they had to wait for dentures.

This brings to mind a woman I treated who was out of work and could not go on a job interview because she was missing her two front teeth. She was a survivor of domestic abuse, and I met her through the Give Back a Smile program, which is run by the American Academy of Cosmetic Dentistry's Charitable Foundation. It is an awesome program that pairs survivors of domestic abuse or sexual violence who have dental injuries with volunteer dentists who donate their time and services. This patient was not only missing her front teeth; she had several other teeth that were off in the gum line, and she'd lost additional teeth due to facial trauma. I jumped at the chance to volunteer and help this woman, and after working out a treatment plan, my wife, Lyndsay, volunteered to do the extractions. I then restored some teeth and replaced others with two removable partial dentures. The result was life changing for the patient.

This woman, who had endured brutal abuse and had a very rough life, had been unable to provide for her children because she couldn't interview for a job. People doing the hiring won't admit it, but if they have two job candidates they're interviewing who have the exact same qualifications, the one who has a good smile will most likely be hired over the one with no front teeth. This is especially true if the job is in customer service or in view of the public. It's sad and unfair, but it happens all the time. In the case of our domestic abuse survivor, once we were finished, she had a healthy mouth, a beautiful smile, and the confidence to go out and interview for any kind of job she wanted. She ended up getting a position as a cashier, a job she most likely would not have been hired for without her teeth. All of this happened because of the Give Back a Smile program, which started in 1999 and has since restored the smiles of more than eighteen hundred people!

When I do volunteer dentistry, I get a lot of cooperation from colleagues and the labs I work with; everyone is eager to jump in and lend a hand. People really do want to help, and many of us who feel blessed to be in the situations we're in want to give back. Take, for example, a patient of mine who I've treated for about eight years.

She recently came into a lot of money and wanted to do something to help. So, we got together to develop a new charity called A Gifted Smile. We're going to select cases from my patient pool who are either veterans or people who have fallen on hard times and need treatment but can't afford it. This amazing woman is going to fund the charity by donating $20,000 a year for the next ten years to cover supplies, and since I won't be charging my patients, I'm going to really be able to make that money go a long way.

The impact we can have is just phenomenal. We're going to make Fridays a charity day, and my whole team will volunteer their time to get these people taken care of. Having my wife on board is huge, since she will do the surgeries, allowing us to tackle the big cases like full mouth reconstruction and implants. It will have a real impact, since some of these cases can cost $20,000 to $30,000. I'm so excited about this program, and my goal is to make that money and the treatments expand even bigger. I'd love to be able to take this program and expand it to the point that it's all I do for a living. I feel so grateful and blessed to have been given the ability to help people, and it's something I love doing. It just feels like the right thing to do.

Many organizations work to provide dental care for those who can't afford it, and one of the most remarkable ones is the Ben Massell Dental Clinic in Atlanta, Georgia. Over 150 volunteer dentists dedicate their skills to provide no-cost care to Atlantans. It's a huge operation! They have sixteen operatories, including two hygiene rooms, and are fully equipped with the latest technologies, all donated by the dental companies in and around Atlanta. The volunteer dentists come from all disciplines, and the clinic also uses seniors from the Dental College of Georgia, who are required to do a rotation there. Last I checked, the volunteers at the Ben Massell Dental Clinic performed more than twenty thousand dental procedures a year, and all of it was at little or no cost. They treat people in the lowest income brackets—people who literally cannot afford anything dental-wise. Lyndsay and I, along with the other wonderful dentists, do all kinds of things over at the clinic: extractions, root canals, surgeries, and dentures.

Unfortunately, the wait time to get a full or partial set of dentures at the Massell clinic has traditionally been very long, and it used to take up to three years to get them. Yes, that's three years of walking around with no teeth. And this was with the clinic working as fast as it could! Although people can function and survive by just gumming food, it's obviously not an ideal situation. However, about three years ago—about five years after Lyndsay and I began volunteering—the clinic got a new director who was just as passionate as we were about reducing that wait time. But how to do it? The clinic was seeing as many patients as quickly as it could. We put our heads together and came up with a way to modify the process. We streamlined some steps and eliminated any that were unnecessary, and we managed to get that wait time down to one year. Our next goal is to get it down to six months, and in the future … who knows? Wouldn't it be great to have it all done in a day? Well, a guy can dream, can't he? But I don't think it's an impossible dream.

Of course, my dream would be that everyone had access to affordable dental care, and it frustrates me that they don't. I am particularly disappointed by the dental insurance companies, which in my opinion have failed us. The system is broken, and here's just one example of how.

In 1972 when the practice I bought first opened its doors, people with dental insurance typically received about $1,500 of annual coverage. Back then, a crown cost about $50 or $100 at a prosthodontic office. These were the days when an average house cost around $20,000, a car around $3,000. So that's almost fifty years ago. If dental insurance today were tied to inflation, people should have about $10,000 of reimbursement. Guess how much the average maximum annual benefit or coverage limit is in 2020? Yep, it's still around $1,500. Unbelievable. It's such a mess.

The insurance companies don't even reimburse the dentists enough to cover lab costs on some procedures. The only way a dentist could survive using the patient's insurance is to do a ton of procedures. And when you do that, you're doing a disservice to the patients, because there is no time or money for proper treatment. Study after study has shown how important oral health is, yet insurance makes little or no provision for it. While it may seem that a couple of hundred dollars is expensive to repair a medium-size cavity, it is a small percentage of the cost to protect that same tooth with a full crown if the cavity wasn't addressed earlier. The lion's share of major dental work that is both costly and time consuming could be significantly reduced with proper prevention and maintenance. It boggles the mind that the insurance companies don't see this and save themselves money in the long run by helping offset the costs of preventative dental care.

People with useless or no dental insurance can certainly check out local organizations, and depending on their financial situation, they may be able to get some help. One great place to go for care would be a dental college. You can get terrific care there because while you're being treated, a faculty member oversees each and every step. It's significantly less expensive because you're helping the students learn a skill and become expert at their craft. I highly recommend looking into this if you're financially strapped.

In this chapter I've given you some useful information if you or someone you know is in a position where they are missing a lot of teeth and desperately need help. After realizing that it's not okay to ignore missing teeth and accepting that fixing the problem will be life changing, it's time to do your research and get some help. If you're in a financial bind, check out your local charities and organizations; you may be surprised at what you find! See if there's a dental college nearby. Ask around about low-interest or zero-interest loans for dental work. At my office we give our patients as much assistance as we can to help solve their problems, and most dentists would be happy to answer your questions and give advice on what your options are. Don't just ignore the issue; it won't go away on its own. There are a lot of professionals out there who can help you, but you have to take the first step.

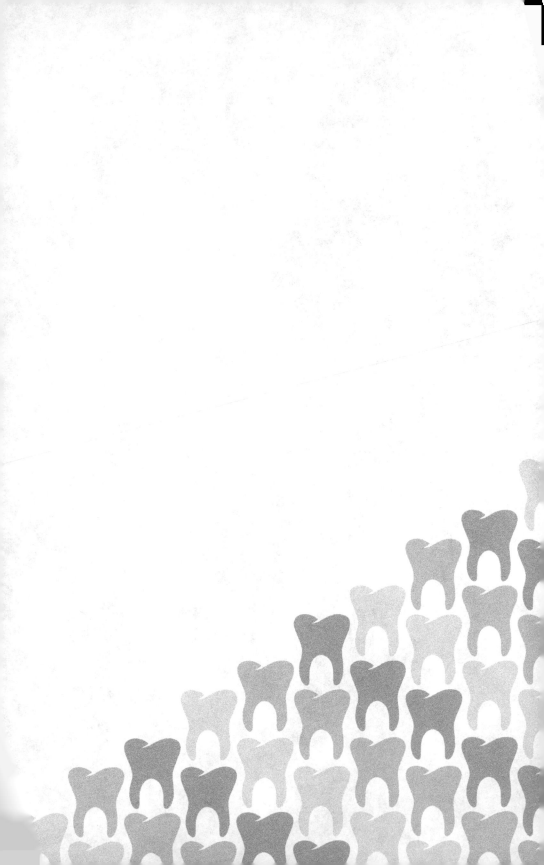

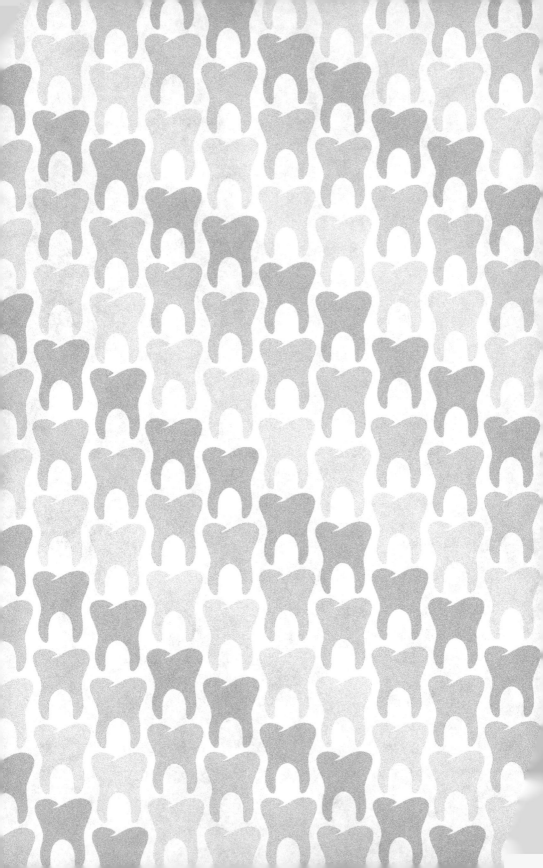

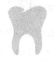

CHAPTER 5

"My Gums Are Very Sensitive When I Brush. What Is That About?"

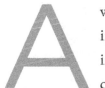while back I had a patient call the office complaining about intense discomfort in her gums. She was in serious distress, and chronic pain was driving her crazy, so she came in for an examination. Now, there are many causes for sensitivity in the gums, but this woman's problem was pretty unique and one I'd never seen before. After examining her under bright lights and using high-powered magnification, I found a red pepper flake wedged between her tooth and gum! It was firmly stuck in there, constantly irritating and burning the tissue. Just think about how that would feel. In no time we were able to pull it out, and the problem was solved. This may seem like a pretty unusual situation, but you'd be surprised how often patients come into the office with mystery pain they think is in their tooth but that turns out to be in the gum tissue.

In my practice we get calls probably twice a week from patients who are experiencing unexplained pain. Sometimes it turns out to be nothing, but other times it requires attention. All too often, a patient feels like there's something stuck in their teeth, and they'll go at it with a toothpick or get overaggressive with floss and end up beating up the gum tissue. By the time they get to us, they've got a big mess. We go in and have a look around. Occasionally the intruder is not obvious, so we'll have to make an incision and pull back the gum tissue to see what's going on.

At least four or five times a year I'll find a popcorn husk that's wedged itself into the tissue. After I remove it, the gum will heal in a hurry. As I mentioned in an earlier chapter, I'm not a fan of popcorn for a number of reasons, and one is those stubborn little husks that love to get trapped in people's teeth. The gum sensitivity and pain caused by these foreign objects are easy to deal with, and I'm always amazed by the body's ability to recover quickly. The healing happens really fast after the foreign object is removed, and the patient's gums feel better right away.

Once in a while we meet patients whose soreness is caused by oral adornments such as tongue bolts, cheek studs, lip rings, and fake gold grills. The grills and piercings can irritate soft gum tissue, which can lead to gum recession, bone loss, and even tooth loss. They can also chip and damage teeth that have previously been restored with crowns or bridgework. If you choose to have oral piercings or use removable grilles, the responsibility will fall on you to visit the dentist more often for checkups and to pay close attention to your oral hygiene.

Occasionally we will have patients come in suffering from sore gums, and after we ask them a few questions, they'll sheepishly admit that the soreness could possibly, *just maybe*, have been caused by their creative use of a household object in an attempt to remove something that's stuck in their teeth. I mentioned the problems caused by overenthusiastically flossing or probing with a toothpick, so you can imagine the trauma resulting from poking around with a paper clip, a ball point pen, or a pencil. How about a key? Or the edge of a stiff piece of cardboard? I cringe just thinking of the damage I've seen from people poking and probing. I do understand there are few things that will drive you up the wall faster than having something stuck between your teeth, but I implore you to give your dentist a call if a careful attempt with some floss, a good rinse, and a careful brushing don't do the trick.

Sometimes the soreness will be caused by the foods people eat, so even if there's nothing caught between the teeth, they might have traumatized the tissue. One of the more interesting things I've seen more than once is damage caused by nacho chips. Because the chip has sharp edges, a miscalculation in biting into one can lacerate the gum. Yes, ouch! Chicken bones are also familiar culprits, and they can act like little daggers, causing nasty cuts. And don't forget about olive pits. I've seen some humdingers of injuries caused by these. Gum tissue is very delicate, so try to remember to be extra vigilant about what goes into your mouth. If you've cut your gums up, give your dentist a call, and even if you did it trying to pry something out from between your teeth using a finishing nail (not recommended, by the way), we promise we won't judge.

Foreign objects aside, another of the most common reasons for gum sensitivity is gingivitis, which is an inflammation of the gum tissue. Gingivitis is very common, and almost everyone has some degree of gum inflammation at some point. The nice thing is that it's completely reversible. Since it's just a swelling, it can be managed with proper home care and dental checkups. However, it absolutely, positively has to be taken seriously, because it is the early stage of periodontal disease, and if it's left unchecked, it will get worse and can lead to tooth loss.

Gingivitis is caused by a bacterial infection in the gums, and there are a few things that will put you at higher risk: poor oral hygiene, smoking, hormonal changes, prescription drugs, old age, and poor nutrition. All these risk factors can allow bacteria in your mouth to get out of control and cause damage.

Did you know that several hundred types of these microscopic organisms can be found in the human mouth? When everything is going well, they live in harmony, but when the balance is disrupted, problems can occur, and harmful bacteria can start to make mischief. The mouth has countless nooks and crannies where these damaging bacteria can take up residence and cause all kinds of trouble—some of it serious. Unfortunately, we inherit some of these bacteria from our parents, so it may be out of our control. When I have a patient tell me his parents and grandparents all had dentures before they were thirty, there's a good chance that patient has a certain type of bacteria in their mouth. If it's not carefully managed, they're going to most likely end up losing their teeth. Different strains of bacteria in your mouth can affect your oral health in a few ways.

One strain of bacteria can be very aggressive toward your teeth and can cause you to develop cavities easily, even if you brush, floss, and stay away from sugary foods. Your teeth are going to be more prone to attack by the bacteria in your mouth. Another strain can attack the bone and the gum tissue around teeth, causing periodontal disease. Patients with an abundance of this type of bacteria may have no cavities and practice good oral care, but for whatever reason, those bacteria attack the bone and eventually a patient will lose the bone, then the tissue, then the teeth. It's almost unbelievable that someone could have no decay and no breakdown but have this unpleasant strain of bacteria that aggressively attacks healthy bone and tissue. Those people are very unlucky and will struggle to keep their teeth healthy for a lifetime. Incredibly, it could be even worse.

Some unlucky folks have both the periodontal disease–causing bacteria *and* the cavity-causing bacteria at the same time. These patients will also struggle despite their best efforts at oral care and prevention. A few lucky people never get cavities or experience tooth loss even if they pay little attention to good oral care and consume tons of sugar. This is a rare subset of the population, but such people do exist. Pretty much everyone falls into one of the categories I mentioned, and it really has to do with the specific type of bacteria in your mouth.

One rather disturbing thing researchers have found is that you can transfer the bacteria that causes periodontal disease to a baby through your saliva. So, if someone has periodontal disease and their saliva makes its way into a baby's mouth, that baby can develop the disease. This transfer can happen even before the baby has teeth. Since babies put just about everything in their mouths, this can happen by kissing them on the hands or face or by sharing a spoon with them. Before you know it, the bacteria makes its way into the baby's mouth. I recommend being vigilant when allowing people to kiss your infant. It could possibly set them up for a lifetime of periodontal disease.

The population of bacteria in the mouth has been studied for a long time, and one area that is of great interest to dental professionals is the idea of changing the flora in people's mouths. If researchers can figure out a way to get the good bacteria in and keep the bad bacteria out, it could be the next big thing in periodontics. Again, this comes back to prevention. How can we prevent periodontitis and tooth loss? Traditionally, the dental industry as a whole has been very reactive. You have a toothache; you come to see me; I fix it or remove it. In the medical profession, they don't wait until your arm falls off, right?

They try to catch things early, to prevent them from happening or getting worse. Dentistry is really starting to focus on training regular people—people just like you—to prevent bad things from happening by educating them about what is normal and what is abnormal in their mouths.

What it boils down to is that if you neglect your oral care, you're going to have problems unless you're one of the very rare people who get away with paying no attention to oral health. If your gums are sore, it's a good idea to find out why, since (as I mentioned, and it's worth repeating) gingivitis is reversible, but if left untreated, you're going to end up with much bigger issues.

What it boils down to is that if you neglect your oral care, you're going to have problems.

Gingivitis leads to minor periodontitis and then on to aggressive or severe periodontitis. When I use the word "aggressive," I'm not exaggerating. You can start losing bone at an alarming rate and get to the point where your teeth literally fall out. You don't want that to happen, and neither do I.

Dentists—and periodontists in particular—are dedicated to saving your teeth. When I work up treatment plans for patients, I always consult my periodontist (who also happens to be my wife). Lyndsay will have a look and do a full evaluation to let me know if the teeth are stable, free of infection, or at risk in some way. The last thing I want to do is have someone undergo an involved treatment, have everything look great, and then have their teeth start failing within a year or two. I want to make sure that, from a periodontal standpoint, the framework and foundation are stable so I can start my work to rebuild. You have to have a healthy mouth before you start putting in implants and bridges. Unfortunately, there are times when we just can't save teeth, but as I said, we're committed to having you keep as many of your natural teeth as possible.

If I may, I'd like to say a few more words about periodontists, since they really are such an integral part of the dental team. Periodontists can work wonders when it comes to helping patients hang on to their own teeth, stopping bone loss, and building bone back up. They can perform procedures that many general dentists don't feel comfortable performing. For example, if you've got an impressive buildup of calculus (tartar) underneath the gum tissue, the periodontist has a great way of getting rid of it. After numbing the area, they will move the gum tissue aside, clean that whole tooth surface, and close the tissue back over. It's a procedure that can help stop bone loss, like hitting the pause button to slow it down. By pausing that bone loss, you can maintain the bone levels that are necessary for the jaw to support your teeth. If there is advanced bone loss, periodontists can actually graft bone—essentially growing new bone for an implant to be placed in. Periodontists can also modify the architecture of the gum tissue, which can be a life changer for someone with a "gummy" smile. Some people are bothered by the amount of gum that shows when they smile, and your friendly periodontist can help with that.

Some of the work done by the periodontist can technically be done by a general dentist, since a dental school graduate has been trained in most areas of dentistry. Theoretically, on day one after you graduate, you are legally allowed to pull teeth, place implants, install braces, and do root canals—the whole shebang. But specialties have been developed to enable a dentist to focus on very specific aspects of care. These specialists have extra training and become highly skilled at what they do. I firmly believe in letting specialists do their thing. There's no way I'm going to do as good a job as someone who has had extensive training and practice. I tell my patients to think of it this way: if you buy an expensive car, you can take it to any body shop and they will probably fix it just fine. But wouldn't you want to take that valuable car to someone who specializes in the brand? I know I would.

I hope I've driven home the importance of paying attention to what's going on with your gums. If they're sore, there's a reason, and it could be as simple as having a red pepper flake stuck between your tooth and gum. It could also signal something more serious that could put you at risk for losing teeth. If you've scraped your gum with the sharp edge of a nacho chip, it will most likely heal on its own. If you've broken off the tip of a toothpick or the lead from a pencil while digging away at something stuck in your teeth, give your dentist a call. That little intruder is most likely not going to come out on its own, and it could actually cause an infection. If your gums are sore for no reason and you can't figure it out on your own, let us help. It could be a simple case of gingivitis, and we can fix that up and prevent it from turning into a full-blown case of periodontitis. You might be one of those people who are unlucky enough to have bacteria attacking your gums. If that's the case, you'll need diligent care to prevent tooth loss, but you can't do it on your own. We are here to help, and we'll figure out the best solution for you and prevent you from experiencing a dental disaster.

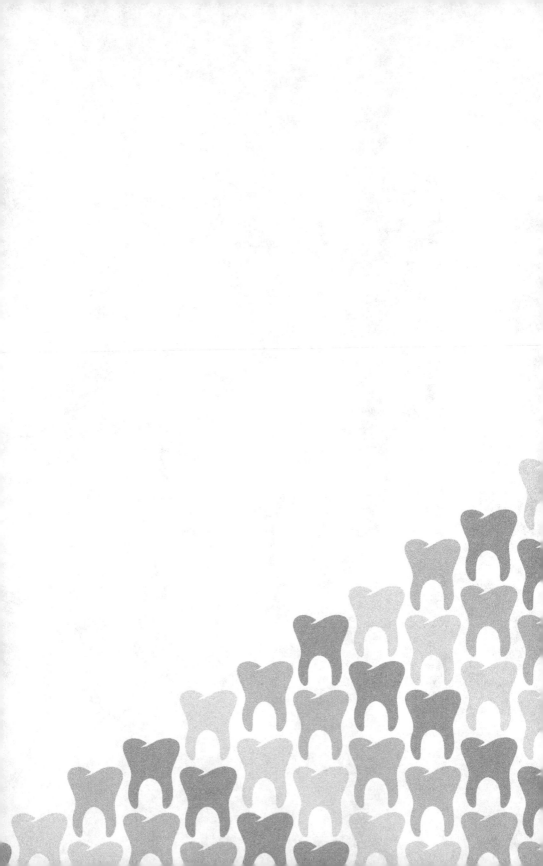

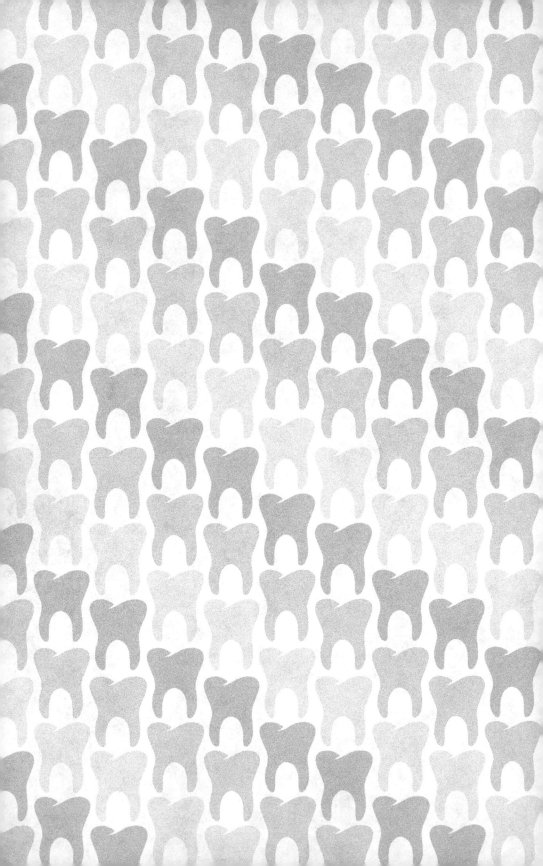

CHAPTER 6

Disasters in Dentistry

ood oral health depends on you and on the dental professionals you choose. You can have the best dentist in the world, but if you don't have a great home routine to care for your teeth and gums, you are putting yourself at risk for cavities and gum disease. Conversely, you can take great care of your mouth, but if you are not careful about the dental services you use, you're asking for trouble. We've had to rescue a significant number of cases where the patient ran into what I call a dental bad actor.

A case in point: I had a patient come in who had several implants done in Costa Rica at a fraction of the cost of doing them in the States. I'm sure she figured it was a great idea; she would save money and have a nice vacation to boot. Well, when she came to me a year or so later, she was in really bad shape. The dentist she used in Costa Rica had placed two implants on either side of her front teeth, and both of them ended up failing. He hadn't taken into consideration—or perhaps wasn't aware—that it's essential to use very specific screws and components. There are hundreds of different brands of implants and screws, and you can't just mix and match them. This patient ended up requiring massive bone grafts, tissue surgery, and replacement of the implants. She may have saved a couple of thousand dollars initially, but she ended up spending somewhere between $15,000 and $20,000 to get the repairs done. She was the victim of a dental bad actor. And believe me, they're out there—from insufficiently trained dentists in foreign countries who target people looking for "destination dentistry" to companies who offer services like teeth straightening through the mail. Of course, there are tons of phenomenally skilled dentists in foreign countries, but if you're trying to pinch pennies, you're not going to be searching out the most expensive, best-qualified dentists outside the United States, are you?

Let's think for a minute about saving money on dental work. Does it really make sense, for example, that you could bypass a highly skilled orthodontist and have a mail-order company straighten your teeth for a third of the cost or less with the same results? Not likely. Remember the old adage that warns you "if something sounds too good to be true, it probably is." Be very wary of popular companies that you see advertised online and places like Facebook that promise to straighten your teeth using plastic aligners they send you in the mail. There is no in-person exam or oversight of the procedure, and this can lead to some really bad outcomes. The idea of straightening teeth without an in-person oral exam, comprehensive X-rays, background screening, and continuous oversight is outrageous. It's not just a matter of moving the teeth around to make them look nice. If orthodontics aren't done correctly, and you move teeth too fast and put them in the wrong kind of torque, you can actually burn through the roots. The roots get shortened, and with the introduction of periodontal disease or bone loss, those teeth are going to become mobile and start moving to places they don't belong. The result: you are at serious risk of losing them.

The advertisements and commercials for mail-order orthodontics don't mention any of these serious drawbacks. These shady companies will do things like sell their systems under the category of cosmetics to avoid scrutiny by the Food and Drug Administration. People will see them on television, on the internet, or at their local Walmart and falsely believe that they've been tested and are safe. Wrong. There are lots of things on the shelves that haven't been properly vetted. It's gotten so bad that the American Dental Association sent a complaint letter to the Federal Trade Commission's Bureau of Consumer Protection in 2019. In the letter they voiced their concerns over SmileDirectClub's plastic teeth aligners. They pointed out that the practices of the Club do not meet standards of patient care and expressed concern over the damage that can occur when procedures that should be handled in person by trained professionals are done with no physical meeting between patient and dentist.

So many things need to be monitored during the course of treatment to avoid tooth erosion, gum recession, incorrect bite occlusion, and potential irreparable harm. Would you really want to risk facing a whole mouth reconstruction because you tried to cut corners by using a mail-order dentist? Let's put it another way. If you break your arm, would you go online and order a cast or splint without having that arm examined and x-rayed? Doing that would be just as crazy as ordering plastic teeth straighteners through the mail.

Okay, hopefully I've convinced you to avoid economy destination dentistry and mail-order orthodontics. Find a local dentist, and make an appointment. Does that mean you won't run into trouble? Unfortunately not. As in any field, you will find that not every dental professional can handle every patient's needs. It doesn't necessarily mean they are bad people; they may have just bitten off more than they can chew (pun intended). We inherit a lot of cases where a dentist has gotten in above their head when taking on a patient who needs complicated treatment. One of the reasons this happens has to do with the way dentists are trained.

When you go to dental school, you train in all the different disciplines, and once you graduate you are legally qualified to perform most everything under the scope of dental treatment. The problem with this is that without continuing education in all the areas of dentistry—and they're numerous—you're not going to be at the top of your game, and you might not be able to handle a difficult case. Conversely, if you specialize in one area and do a residency focusing only on one aspect of dentistry, you get really good at it. Remember, I spent three years in my prosthodontic residency focusing solely on restoring and replacing missing or broken teeth. That's a lot of practice! By keeping up your education in a specific area, you can be part of a team that handles even the most complicated cases.

I think it would be beneficial to give you a quick overview of the dental specialties, since there are a number of them and it can get a little confusing. Here are some that are important for you to know:

Oral Surgeon—Practitioners are highly skilled surgeons of the mouth and focus on extracting teeth, bone wrapping, reconstructive surgery, and placing implants.

Periodontist—Like oral surgeons, they perform surgeries of the mouth, but they tend to do more focused microsurgeries. In addition to doing these specialized surgeries on the gums and bone, they also extract teeth, place implants, and do grafts.

Prosthodontist—These specialists repair, replace, and reconstruct broken or missing teeth. They handle the most complicated full mouth reconstructions.

Endodontist—These are the root canal specialists, and although they'll sometimes do other minor surgeries, their focus is on root canals.

Orthodontist—Their specialty is moving teeth using braces. They might work in conjunction with a surgeon to align teeth to get them in the right spot in order to build things around them.

Oral Pathologist—These professionals specialize in diagnosing and treating diseases in the mouth. They detect and manage cancers, lesions, jaw misalignment, and other unhealthy abnormalities.

Pediatric Dentists—These dentists specialize in treating infants and children.

It can be enticing to play the hero by doing a full mouth reconstruction and totally changing someone's life on your own, but unless you really know what you're doing, it's best to work with a team of specialists following a very specific treatment plan. It's important to choose wisely. It's your mouth, and you have a right to know what your dentist plans for you and question whether or not they feel confident handling it all on their own. Knowledge is power, and now that you know, you should feel free to investigate and ask questions about your care.

This leads me to think about the differences between corporate dentistry and the traditional dental practice. You might have noticed these chain dental offices popping up all over the place; that's what I mean by corporate dentistry. They usually have big buildings, and their practices are insurance driven, meaning that to be profitable, they really have to crank out the cases to make money. Unfortunately, you won't always find the most honest practices in these efficiently run but impersonal offices. We've had patients come in telling us stories of being pushed into unnecessary procedures at great expense. I'm not saying all these places are like that, but it's a common theme we see in our practice. Quite often my patients tell me that even though we're a little more expensive, they trust us, and so it's worth the added cost. They know that when they visit us, they'll get the care they need and *only* what they need.

It's your right to ask questions, and if you ever tell a dentist that you want a second opinion and they get upset or frustrated with you, that's a red flag.

It's the same kind of thing as choosing to visit the mom-and-pop hardware store versus the giant home improvement centers. At the smaller stores, the owners are knowledgeable and are there to help you. They might charge a little more, but they would never run the risk of losing your business by selling you things you don't need. At the giant stores, you most likely won't find anyone who knows the inventory well enough to help you buy just what you need, and you may end up loading your cart with unnecessary items. You get the idea.

It's important to remember that the overwhelming majority of dentists, especially those in private practice, are good people and really do want to do right by you. When it comes to private practice dentists, they can sometimes get ahead of themselves and try to plan too much or have cases they're just not equipped to handle on their own. In those instances, they should, and usually do, seek out the help of specialists and make it a team effort. As I mentioned, it's your right to ask questions, and if you ever tell a dentist that you want a second opinion and they get upset or frustrated with you, that's a red flag. Every reputable dentist wants you to be happy with your treatment plan. They want you to understand exactly what is going to happen. I fully welcome any of my patients to ask questions, and I'll even call and make a referral for them to get a second opinion. My main goal is to make them comfortable with me and the work I've planned for them. I hope that after seeking a second opinion, they'll come back to me and say "Sorry, doc. Your plan was right on!" and I can get to work knowing they have faith in me. Fortunately, that's usually what happens.

I've given you a lot of information here, so let me summarize some widespread dental myths:

1. **All dentists are equally competent**. Not true. As in nearly every profession on the planet, you'll have those who are better at what they do than others. Again, the vast majority of us are good, qualified professionals. But you should do your research and learn as much as you can so you can make good decisions. Ask questions; talk to people, and if you are not comfortable with the dentist you've chosen, go somewhere else.

2. **You can save a bundle having the same dental work done in foreign countries that you can have done here at home**. Destination dentistry in places like Costa Rica or Mexico will cost less up front, but you are taking a big gamble. Unless you seek out the most expensive dentists with the best reputations in these foreign countries, you are putting your oral health at risk. You could end up spending way more than you should have when you find yourself with failing dental work, infection, or worse.

3. **You don't need an orthodontist. You can straighten your teeth with a mail-order kit.** No, no, no. I would never recommend doing this. Never. Common sense will tell you that someone who has trained for years to straighten teeth is going to do a much better job than a mail-order company. Yes, it will cost more, but you will avoid the possibility of a whole world of aggravation and expense.

4. **Corporate dentists are no different than private practice dentists.** Even if a chain dentist does competent work, you're never going to get the personal care at a factory-type dental office that you'll get with a private practitioner. Corporate dental practices will often push you to spend money on procedures you don't necessarily need. They won't care about you as an individual the way a small practice will.

5. **Dentists choose this profession to make tons of money.** In the vast majority of cases, this is false. It pains me when I tell a patient they need a crown or some other procedure, and they say something like "Oh, I guess we know who's paying for your new boat," or "Oh, I suppose this will help with your children's college funds." People don't realize how

expensive dentistry is for us. Overhead is huge, lab costs have skyrocketed, and keeping up with the newest technology is far from cheap. In my practice, the staff is deservedly well compensated, and I spend a lot of money on state-of-the-art equipment. Of course, there are dentists who chose this profession thinking that they are going to take a walk on easy street, but in the long run it's just not the way it works.

Before I end this overview of dental bad actors and disasters, I want to mention something that has become increasingly popular in the world of do-it-yourself dentistry: those snap-on veneers that you see advertised just about everywhere online; the ones with names like "Smile-o-Matic" or "X-pressmile." (These aren't their real names, but you get the idea.) The concept is that for a few bucks, you get a do-at-home mold kit to take an impression of your mouth, and after sending it back to the company, you receive a set of veneers that fit over your natural teeth. The mechanics are much the same as for those monster teeth you buy your kids at Halloween, since they slide right over your natural teeth. The veneers are advertised to give you a beautiful smile, boost your confidence, and change your entire life. Yes, well, that's a really cool idea, and certainly these veneers are fine to wear to a party once in a while, but that's not how they're advertising them, and that's not how people are using them.

If you wear these veneers too much, they can push on the gum tissue, put pressure on the teeth, and can actually cause the teeth to start shifting. Even worse, they tend to trap bacteria and food in all the pockets and recesses. If someone puts these in at the beginning of the day and wears them until bedtime, the natural teeth have no opportunity to get a nice saliva rinse. Saliva is nature's way of keeping food, debris, and plaque away from teeth. Without it, the teeth under those veneers are spending the day sitting in a bacteria stew. Finally, by hiding decaying or broken teeth, people run the risk of avoiding a visit to the dentist. "Out of sight, out of mind" thinking is never a good idea in dentistry.

As we conclude our overview of dental disasters, I'd like you to keep a few things in mind. First, it's best to have your dental work done by someone you know has been properly trained and is in a position to be held accountable. Your oral health is just as important as the health of the rest of your body, so you don't want to cut corners and search out the cheapest solution. Not only could you end up injured—you may also have to pay dearly for your choices. I encourage you to do your research before you make such an important decision. Again, if something sounds too good to be true, it probably is. You need a professional to care for your mouth, and dentistry can't be done properly through the mail or online. I urge you to watch out for trendy appliances that promise to give you a beautiful smile. They're fine to use once in a while, but when they prevent you from seeking out the care you need, they become problematic. If you wear them all the time, you are putting the overall health of your mouth at risk. There have been great strides in dental care, especially in the past few decades. Take advantage of them!

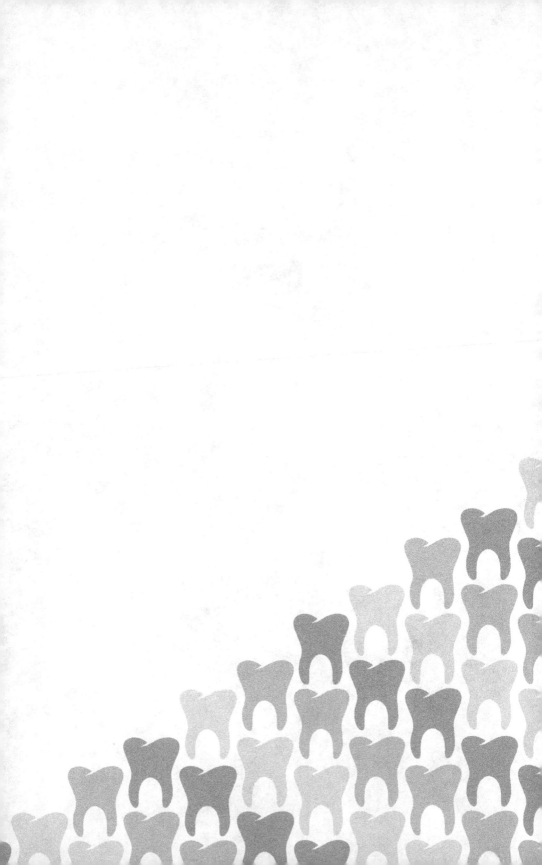

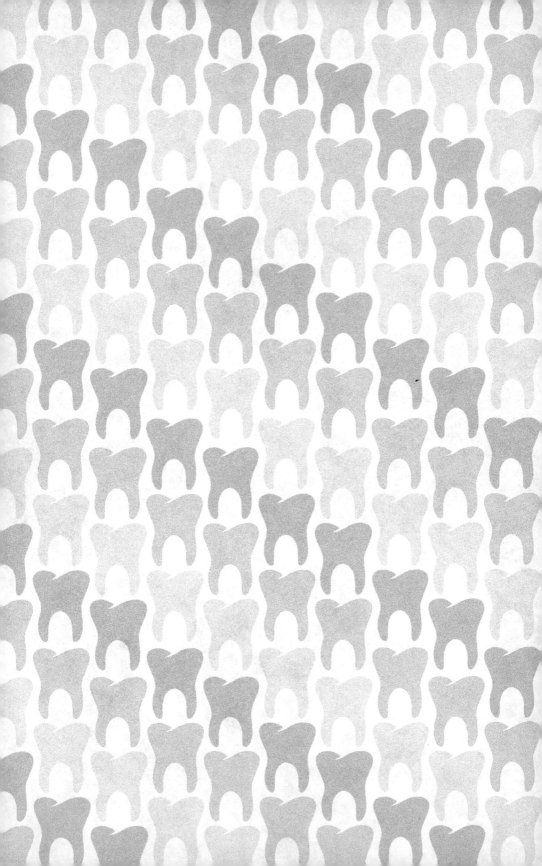

How a Rabbit Leg Revolutionized Dental Prosthetics

H istory is full of examples of accidental discoveries that changed the world, and the usefulness of titanium for dental implants is one of the most compelling. It all began in the 1950s when Swedish orthopedic surgeon and medical researcher Per-Ingvar Brånemark and his team were investigating the way blood flow affects the healing process of bone. For their experiments, they used rabbits as subjects, and to observe the healing, they inserted optical titanium viewing chambers into the animals' legs so they could monitor the process. Once the bone was healed, they attempted to remove the viewing windows and found that the titanium had fused to the bone. The integration of the bone with the titanium was so complete that the viewing windows could not be removed. Brånemark was so intrigued by this discovery that he changed the direction of his work and began investigating how and why the human body tolerated titanium, even coining the word "osseointegration" to describe the process of bone integrating with metal.

Before the discovery of the biocompatibility of titanium and bone, people tried out all kinds of implant materials to replace missing teeth, including pieces of shell or stone, cadaver teeth, gold, and surgical steel. None of these were as successful as titanium. Researchers found that a cylindrical root-form implant made of titanium was the best option, since it allowed the bone cells to grow onto the metal, forming a permanent bond and mimicking the natural root.

When Brånemark's implants first came into the dental mainstream, there was a highly guarded membership of who was allowed to place them in a patient's jaw. The original lectures were given in Sweden, and the restorative doctor had to fly there with a surgeon for instruction directly from Brånemark himself. Brånemark didn't want just anyone to try his technique, and for a time it was a very protected procedure. Nowadays dental implanting is done just about everywhere in the world, and there are hundreds of different implant brands in every shape and size. It's become a huge industry and has continued to evolve.

When I was in dental school during the early 2000s, implants were not very common, and I only did a handful during my four years. However, by the time I got to my residency around 2009, we were doing implants left and right. According to the *Journal of Dental Research*, implant use rose from 0.7 percent in 1999 to 2000 to 5.7 percent in 2015 to 2016.[2] The data suggests that by 2026, usage could be as high as 23 percent, so it's a rapidly growing practice.

---

2   H. W. Elani, J. R. Starr, and G. O. Gallucci et al, "Trends in Dental Implant Use in the U.S., 1999–2016, and Projections to 2026," *Journal of Dental Research* 97, no. 13, August 3, 2018, https://doi.org/10.1177/0022034518792567.

The study also found that the prevalence of implant use was higher among advantaged groups, which translates as "they're expensive." The technology will continue to improve, and competition to manufacture implant components will heat up, but prices probably won't drop very much overall. Implant companies spend a lot of money on research and development, so the costs are high. Lab fees are expensive because the way you have to attach the implants is very meticulous and specific. Any respectful dentist will buy a certain company's attachment piece, the custom piece, and the crown. The customization of the actual tooth that fits over the implant is very intensive and expensive. The tooth has to be matched perfectly to the patient's bite, the shade of the tooth has to be matched, and the size has to be exact. There's a significant amount of administrative and supply cost, which probably won't drop much. Still, if a patient can work out the financing, implants are a great value because they have a high success rate and will most likely last a lifetime.

During my career, I've watched the remarkable evolution of the dental implant, and the technology just keeps getting better and better. Originally the top part of the implant post was flat and had a small knob sticking up that the crown was attached to with a screw. All the force was retained by that little, tiny dental screw, and we had problems with the screws loosening over time. Every couple of years we had to have the patient come in so we could tighten the screw. It wasn't the end of the world, but we all knew it could be better. Researchers eventually developed an internal technology where the implant piece goes inside so it engages a lot more metal on metal, and most of the force is transmitted to the implant and not the screw itself. They've also developed all kinds of new coatings to put on the outside of the implant that encourage bone growth and attachment, resulting in better health to the whole area. Overall, the technology is really outstanding when you consider how far it's come in the past few decades.

I feel blessed to be living during a time when dental technology is evolving at such a rapid rate, and I always try to keep up with the latest discoveries. Dentists are required to take twenty hours of continuing education a year, but that's really a drop in the bucket for what you need to stay current. Dentistry does an amazing job of providing continuing education opportunities, and I take advantage of as many as I can. (I told you I was a dental geek.) I find all the new technology fascinating and want to learn as much as possible. Although many of the techniques in dentistry remain the same, the materials and diagnostic tools have gotten much better, resulting in not only increased success of procedures but a more patient-friendly experience.

Materials and diagnostic tools have gotten much better, resulting in not only increased success of procedures but a more patient-friendly experience.

Let me tell you a little about the evolution of materials used to make crowns. Traditionally, layered porcelain was used to create crowns, and although it's a wonderful material, practitioners found that using ceramic or zirconia is more beneficial. One of the problems with the old porcelain crowns is that they are not as compatible with existing teeth. If, for example, you have porcelain crowns on the top and natural teeth on the bottom, the porcelain acts as an abrasive and is quite aggressive on your real teeth, wearing them down much faster. Ceramic and zirconia are very lifelike and extremely durable with the added benefit of wearing down at about the same rate as enamel, so there's great compatibility.

Gold is also quite compatible with existing teeth since it's a soft metal. It's malleable enough to get into all the nooks and crannies and wears down at about the same rate as enamel. I have many patients who had gold work done in the seventies, and it's held up wonderfully and looks phenomenal. Of course, most patients will prefer a crown that blends in with their existing teeth, so we primarily use ceramic and zirconia for crowns.

The materials used to make full or partial dentures have also changed significantly since humans began creating sets of false teeth using ivory, wood, or animal teeth thousands of years ago. Early prosthetics were heavy, uncomfortable, and easily broken. If you ever get a chance, take a look at the set of George Washington's dentures on display at Mount Vernon or on their website. It's a torturous-looking contraption made of wires, springs, metal, and an assortment of teeth taken from cows, horses, and people. (No, George's teeth were not made of wood.) The materials we now use for dentures, specifically the acrylics, are strong, lifelike, and stain resistant. They have the bonus of possessing antibacterial qualities, which is fantastic. They're comfortable and functional and look quite natural. Some patients opt for ceramic dentures, but personally I don't use them. Ceramics are much heavier, so it's harder to maintain the retention, and they tend to slip out of place and clack against each other. So even if you have a well-fitting denture, the weight of it can cause problems and embarrassment for the patient.

In the not-too-distant past, the chance that a denture patient would have problems that might lead to embarrassment was much higher than it is now. Before, if you had a full set of dentures, you had to rely on suction and the fit of the prosthetic to the tissue. Dentures easily slid around or occasionally fell out. Now we can put implants into the jaw, which we can then attach the denture to, or we can create a precisely fitted traditional set of dentures. The implant-supported dentures are a great innovation in that they are comfortable, functional, and natural looking. We insert implants into the upper and lower jaw, and we add four little snaps, so when you put your dentures in, they securely snap into place. They are super secure; in fact, they can be a little too secure, so we are able to modify how easily they snap in and out of place.

We've had to change the way we do things with the snap-in dentures because inevitably I'd get a call from a patient who had just gotten their new dentures that day and couldn't get them out that night. "Doc, I've spent years having my teeth fall out when I talk or chew, and now I can't get them out!" If you think about it, it's a good problem to have, but we don't want anyone struggling at night to remove dentures, and we certainly don't want them left in. We now start with a little less retention and make it stronger if needed. These implant dentures are a really terrific innovation and can also be life changing.

A few years ago, I had a patient who loved to play the trombone. He had lost all his teeth when he was young, and although he had dentures, he found that they affected his performance on the trombone. With his dentures in he was constantly having to shift and maneuver his lips to keep his teeth in place. It was a struggle, a real juggling act. When he was alone, he played without his teeth, and the music sounded much better since he didn't have to deal with slipping dentures. This caused him a lot of sadness and frustration, since he took great pride in his musical performances, but his self-consciousness prevented him from playing in public without his teeth. But don't worry, this story has a happy ending, because we got him all fixed up with snap-in dentures that allowed him to play freely without worrying about embarrassing accidents. He was thrilled to be able to give his best performances with his beautiful teeth in place.

Another musical patient of mine is one of the sweetest ladies I've ever met, and I'm happy to say we were able to help her also. She has a condition called scleroderma, which caused the muscles in and around her mouth to tighten, leading to her having a very tiny mouth opening and a few other oral issues. Since she had such a small mouth opening, the process of making her dentures became very difficult because she basically needed a miniature denture just to fit into her mouth. Once it was in, there wasn't much real estate to grab onto to make it stable. She'd had multiple sets of dentures made in the past and had never been happy with the results. This affected her ability to perform in her church choir, and although she could sing with the group, she was never able to take a starring role because she constantly kept her hand near her mouth in case her dentures slipped or fell out. When she came to us, we did a thorough examination and prepared a treatment plan. We worked with an oral surgeon, did some modifications on her ridge, and made her a smaller snap-in denture, which never would have worked without the implants. Afterward she was able to sing and speak to her heart's content. She became much more involved in her church and was able to belt out her songs, arms waving and not a care in the world. It was really awesome to see her transformation and give her the ability to participate in something she was passionate about.

Speaking of passion, I'd like to mention how ill-fitting dentures can have an effect on intimate relationships. Imagine how intimidating it would be to kiss someone and worry that your dentures are going to fall out. I've heard a lot of stories of people whose personal lives have been affected by the condition of their mouths; it's not unusual for people to shy away from making intimate connections because of their fear of having dentures slip or fall out. With all the wonderful solutions I've talked about, there is no reason for people to live this way anymore. Even if they don't have a tooth left in their mouths, we can fix them up and provide them with secure, natural-looking dentures that allow them to follow their dreams and make personal connections without fear.

We are living in a time when the technology available for dentistry is unparalleled in history. We've got titanium implants that bond with bone and function in much the same way as a natural tooth root, lightweight and durable materials that look exactly like real teeth, and state-of-the-art methods for diagnosis and treatment planning. The choices available to patients are many, and there are skilled practitioners who can literally change people's lives with their artistry. Knowledge is power, and I hope that now you are aware of the many solutions available for just about any kind of dental issue. As the technology continues to develop, I'm sure there will be even more choices that will enable people to have a fully functioning, healthy mouth.

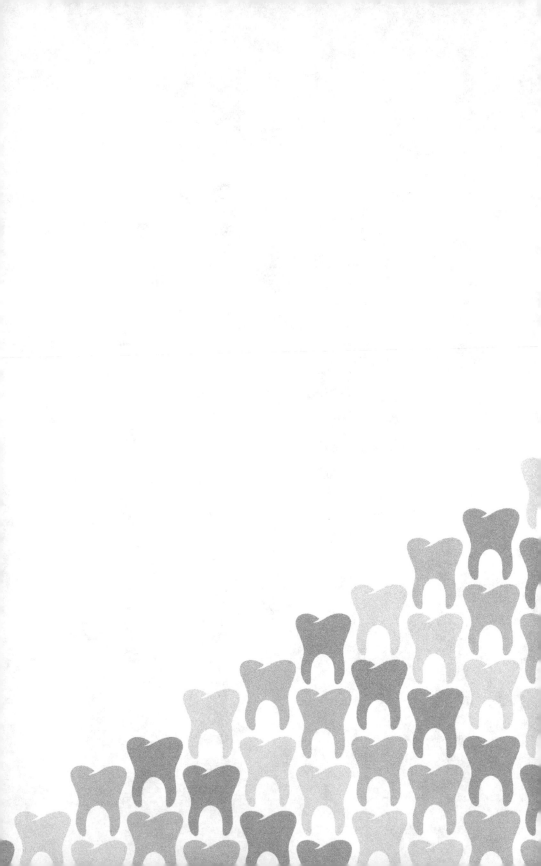

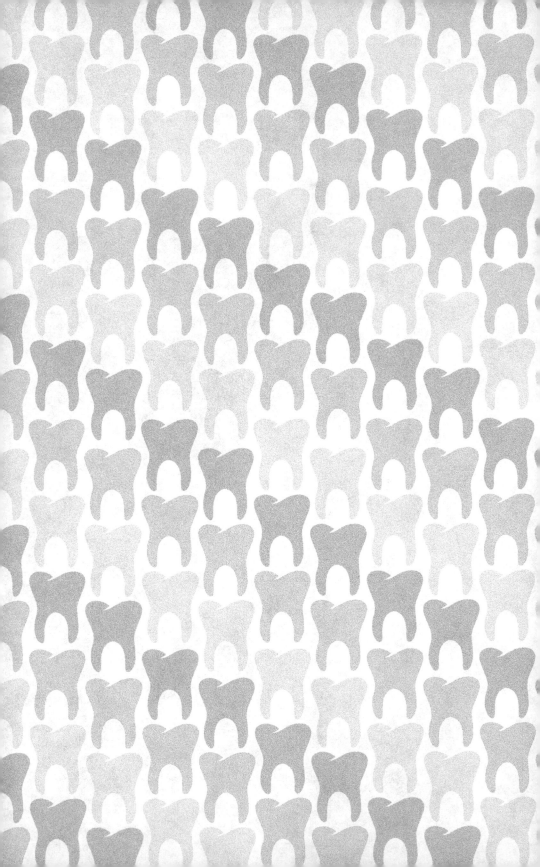

CHAPTER 8

"I Have a New Set of Implants, So Now I Have Unbreakable Bionic Teeth"

B y now you know how much I love dental technology, from diagnostics to treatments. Modern materials are truly awe inspiring in their ability to mimic Mother Nature, especially when it comes to the materials used to create false teeth. That being said, it's still important to respect the dental work and treat it with care. There are no such things as truly "bionic" teeth.

When Lyndsay and I were doing our residencies in the army,

There are no such things as truly "bionic" teeth.

we had a middle-aged sergeant major come in for some extensive work. After removing several nonviable teeth, we put three implants on the top and three on the bottom toward the back of his mouth. Once the permanent crowns were put in, everything looked perfect, and he was good to go. However, without missing a beat, this guy would come in every two months or so with a fractured crown or a broken implant. Lyndsay and I were mystified trying to figure out what was going on with this man until we did a little questioning and found out that he loved to chew on chicken bones. He would take the chicken wings and drumsticks, and instead of biting the meat off, he would chew the whole thing, bones included. Since implants have no nerves in them, he didn't have any perception of how hard he was chewing and how damaging it was. He kept eating his chicken bones and breaking his crowns and implants until we had a little talk with him. We stressed the fact that although his implants and crowns were very sturdy, they needed to be cared for a little more delicately. No more chicken bones.

After dealing with our chicken bone guy and, believe it or not, a college kid who loved to show off his party trick of opening beer bottles with his implant crown (yeah, he cracked it), we revamped our patient instructions to further stress that implants and crowns needed to be cared for just like you would care for regular teeth. Some people are under the mistaken impression that once they get implants, they don't have to brush their teeth regularly. This is incorrect and can lead to peri-implantitis, a disease that causes inflammation around the implant and can lead to bone loss and tissue damage.

Of course, we had always instructed patients to floss and brush, but we expanded that a bit to cover more specific hazards to the newly implanted teeth. It's also important for patients to be educated on the healing process, since the more they understand about exactly what is happening, the more likely they are to tread lightly when it comes to their implants. It takes a good three to four months for the implant to bond with the bone, so care should be taken until that happens. I like to explain to patients that an implant crown is basically a three-part stack, almost like an ice cream cone with two scoops. First you have the titanium screw that goes directly into the bone. On top of that you have the custom-made piece that is screwed into the implant and sticks above the gum tissue, resembling a miniature tooth. Finally, you have the crown—the piece that looks like a real tooth—that goes on top. When we place the implant into the jawbone, the natural bone cells around it begin to die off and are replaced by new bone. The new bone is actually what grows onto and fuses with the metal. If you are not careful and jostle the implant at this vulnerable time, the new cells won't be able to grow, and the old cells won't be able to hold it anymore. That's when you get implant failure. So, it's really important to baby that implant for three or four months, and we tell patients that if they can't cut their food using just a fork, don't eat it until the implant has fully healed. Once everything is healed up, it's still important to be cautious (i.e., don't chew chicken bones) to avoid fractures or implant failure. I don't want to scare anyone into thinking that during the healing period they have to eat only oatmeal and yogurt. On the contrary, life should remain pretty much the same for a patient in the three or four months post surgery. They just have to be a little more cautious. The more careful they are, the better the bond will be, and the probability for long-term success of the implant will increase.

One of the biggest reasons for the success of dental implants is the materials used to make the various components. The implants themselves (the part we put into the bone) are made of commercially pure titanium. As Dr. Brånemark discovered, titanium is easily accepted by the human body and allows bone to bond to it. We're also starting to get into using zirconia implants, zirconia being a strong white metal

TEETH AREN'T JUST FOR SMILING

that has consistent quality and stability. Because of its biocompatibility with the human body, zirconia is the material of choice for things like hip joints or femoral ball joints. It is quite cutting edge and is a great option for patients who have a titanium allergy (pretty rare) or very thin bone. Before zirconia was discovered as an option for dental implants, it was either titanium or nothing, so we're lucky to have it.

The piece that attaches to the screw installed in the bone (remember our ice cream cone analogy?) is usually made of titanium, gold, or zirconia, which are all highly biocompatible. Options for the crown itself are many: gold, zirconia, ceramic, porcelain, or some combination of those. These materials have evolved to the point where they're very strong and wear at the same rate as the opposing teeth. They are also able to handle the extremely harsh environment of the mouth. If you factor in the acidic component of the human mouth, add the foods you eat, the saliva, and the masticatory cycle (how much you chew and with how much force), it's pretty amazing that we've got materials we can put in your mouth that will last a lifetime without damaging existing teeth. They're super strong, esthetic, and make for long-lasting implants.

Of course, it's still important for implant patients to visit the dentist regularly. We need to monitor the health of the tissue around the implant because even the most successful implant loses a little bone each year, and long-term implants need to be monitored closely just to be sure all is well. Even people who have great hygiene habits may have a "brushing blind spot" or an area that they consistently miss with a toothbrush. This can cause inflammation, so it's best to visit a hygienist who can get into all the little nooks and crannies. We have great ultrasonic scalers and other devices that will keep everything in your mouth in good shape. Even my patients who have dentures and/or only a few natural teeth come visit every six months. This gives us a chance to check the tissue health, do an oral cancer screening, and make sure everything is going well inside the mouth. As I mentioned before, prevention is the key.

I've told you a lot about the mechanics of putting in a dental implant and described the healing process, so now I'd like to talk about one more thing that is likely on your mind: pain. As I mentioned earlier in the book, many people avoid the dentist because of their fear of pain.

I've had patients tell me that in their opinion, nothing is worse than dental pain. Not childbirth, kidney stones, or even exploding appendixes. Their fear runs that deep. I am very aware of patient fear—I truly am—and I don't want anyone to be afraid of me. When we talk about the scary-sounding procedure of installing implants, I want to reassure you that having a dentist drill into your bone to screw a piece of metal into your jaw sounds much, *much* worse than it really is.

First of all, bone has no nerves, so you can stop thinking, "Uh-oh. This guy is going to be drilling a hole in my jaw and screwing in a piece of metal—that's got to hurt!" Please don't worry. Dental anesthetics have come such a long way, and we have the ability to use modern topicals and techniques that cause patients little discomfort. Most people barely feel the injection!

We won't be strapping you down and drilling away with no anesthetic, I promise. Sadly, I have had patients who have experienced just this kind of thing when they were young, and it's horrible and traumatic. It sets them up for an entire lifetime of dental anxiety. It's just not that way anymore. I can't speak for every dentist, but I assure you that at my practice and at most responsible dental offices, we are focused on patient care and comfort. We want everybody to love coming to see us and not have the anxiety that it's going to be some hellish scene from a torture movie.

You will be completely numb for the procedure, and you'll probably be sore for a while when it's over. I have patients fall asleep in my dental chair all the time while I'm working on them, and no, I'm not kidding. I take this as a huge compliment that they are comfortable enough with us that they can actually fall asleep while we are working on their mouths. The chairs we have at my practice are extremely comfortable, plus we use soothing colors and calming music to create a tranquil and friendly atmosphere. Our intense efforts to put our patients at ease allows them to relax, some of them to the point where they just nod off. And I'm not talking about a medically induced sleep!

This is a very rewarding experience for me, as it demonstrates a high level of trust from my patients. It makes me happy when patients tell me that a visit to the dentist is so much better than it used to be.

Of course, some patients are extremely anxious, so no amount of calming music or soft colors will put them at ease, and for them we have nitrous gas and antianxiety medications that can help a lot.

Still hesitant? Well, if you're one of those people who just can't handle the experience at all, there is the option of sedation dentistry, where you'll be knocked out for the whole time. You won't know a thing, and by the time you wake up, you're good to go. You won't remember the process at all.

As for postoperative pain, drilling into the bone and installing the implant causes about the same soreness as having a tooth extracted. Your gum tissue will be irritated for a few days, but it's not going to be too bad, trust me. When I do big cases on a Friday, my patients will be back to work on Monday feeling pretty good. The rest of the three or four months are spent in a state of passive healing, and you won't feel much of anything from the procedure.

In cases where there are multiple extractions, there will be more widespread postoperative pain and swelling, but the pain is not severe or unbearable. The nice thing is that if we install the same-day prosthetics, they act kind of like a fancy bandage that looks and functions like teeth and at the same time protects the surgical site. If we don't immediately attach the teeth to the implant, we'll use a temporary denture that protects the extraction site.

Finally, if you're worried about the esthetics, one of my goals in planning the procedure and foreseeing the healing process is to never have a patient go without their front teeth. I think everyone has a fear that they're going to wake up and have no front teeth, and it will be emotionally bankrupting, so we always make a plan to at least give patients a temporary solution.

To recap, there are no indestructible teeth, and even the best of modern-day implants need to be handled with care. The three to four months following implantation are the most crucial, and after that you're home free—but that doesn't mean you can chew bones or pop open beer bottles with your new teeth. Treat them with respect, and they'll reward you with a lifetime of service.

Yes, the process of implantation can be complicated, but it is not overly painful, and there

The process of implantation can be complicated, but it is not overly painful, and there is no reason to feel anxious about it.

is no reason to feel anxious about it. Dental practices put a lot of time and research into improving the patient experience, and if you haven't been to a dental office in years, you'll be pleasantly surprised when you visit. We're here to put you at ease and give you the best patient experience possible. And although we can't give you bionic teeth, we can give you natural-looking, functional teeth that will last for many years.

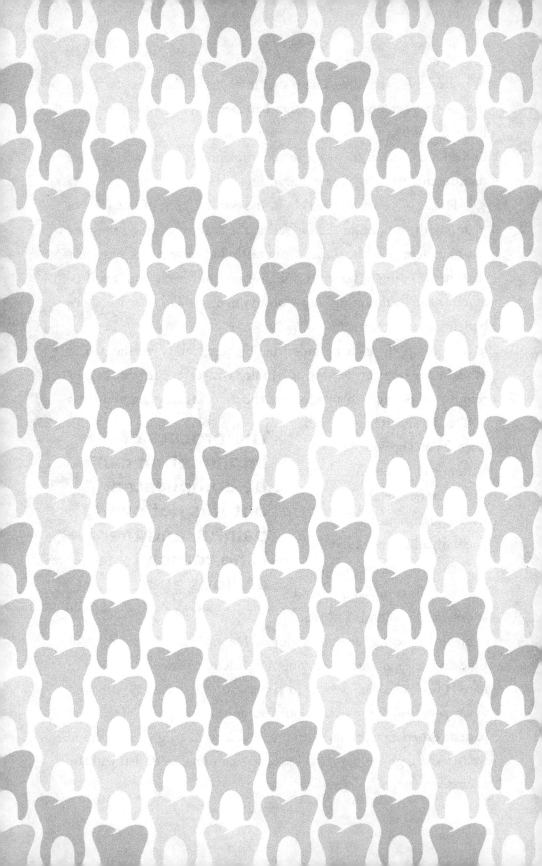

More Lasers, Less Goop: The Teeth of the Future

I magine a world where you could enter a dentist's office, have a digital scan done of your broken or compromised tooth, and within an hour and a half your dentist will have installed a custom-created, brand-new ceramic tooth for you. No goopy mouth impressions to wait to set up, no temporary crown, no return visit three weeks later. None of that. Sounds like something out of a science fiction story, right? Would you be surprised to know that this is something we do at my practice *all the time*? We use a computer-aided design and milling system to create CEREC (Chairside Economical Restoration of Esthetic Ceramics) crowns, and the system is at the forefront of single-visit dental restorations.

In the past, patients had to endure sitting for a length of time with a mouthful of impression material, a clay-like goop that caused a lot of people to choke and gag. It had a disagreeable taste, a clay-like consistency, and could stain clothing, making for an overall unpleasant experience for most folks. I have firsthand knowledge of the entire distasteful process since I spent nearly every Friday of my first year in residency learning the old techniques and historical materials used in the past for doing mouth impressions. Since the residents practiced on each other, I spent more than my fair share of time sitting in a chair with a mouthful of impression goop, waiting for it to set up.

Happily, we've gotten to the point where we can do a lot of this digitally now. We can scan the mouth or a specific tooth, send the scan to a lab, and have them prepare a crown, or, as is the case with my practice, we can use the CEREC system right in the office. Basically, I will do the scan, design the crown, mill it out of a solid block of ceramic, and then bond it in place. The patient can watch the whole process, and even for someone who isn't a dental enthusiast, it's fascinating to see. I've got the computers and the milling unit right in my office.

The computer is state of the art and can calculate and design a very accurate replica of a tooth. It looks at adjacent and opposing teeth and can figure out the ideal tooth shaped just for the patient's mouth. The milling machine then takes the digital information, and using a block of ceramic, it whittles it down to the exact specifications, resulting in a tooth-colored ceramic crown that's designed to fit perfectly in your mouth. Since I'm a bit of a perfectionist, I like to tinker with it even further to customize it. If it's not just the right shape, the patient's tongue is going to constantly feel around for it, and it will drive them crazy. All in all, the process is a very pleasant and stress-free experience for the patient and saves considerable time in dental restoration. Compare this process to my having a patient come in so I can take an impression, install a temporary crown, and have them return in three weeks when the new crown is ready. Imagine the convenience of a system like this if you crack a tooth when you're on vacation. Single-visit dental restoration is certainly a game changer.

As wonderful as the system is, CEREC is expensive for a dental practice, so they may not show up in the mainstream for a while because of the cost. My newest unit and mill were around $150,000, and there are additional costs for supplies. Despite this, at my practice we are able to charge the same price for CEREC as for lab-fabricated ceramic, gold, or zirconium crowns because the lab fees and associated costs are significantly lower when I make the crown in my office. I'm also able to eliminate a non-revenue-producing appointment, since the old way required a second appointment to seat the crown. The decreased lab fees and freed-up appointments in my schedule have allowed me to cover the cost of financing the CEREC system. I also feel that providing same-day service to the patient is a fantastic customer benefit that increases patient satisfaction and improves the likelihood that the patient will refer family and friends to our office for the same incredible care.

I try to make the whole process as easy on the patient as possible and enable them to choose the best material for a specific tooth in their mouth without cost playing a role in their decision, so I charge the exact same price for ceramic and gold crowns despite their vastly different lab costs. When I create a CEREC crown, I use the same materials, usually a ceramic called lithium disilicate, that my lab would use if I ordered it from them. There's no compromise in strength, esthetics, or integrity; it just saves the patient from having to wear a temporary crown and come for a second visit.

There is, however, a very steep learning curve when it comes to the CEREC software and equipment, so that will limit the number of practices that can use it until they get the training. I was lucky to have been able to train on this technology when I was in the army, where I could spend several hours with a patient to learn and study the techniques. In private practice, if you spend three hours working on a crown for one patient, you're not going to survive, especially if you factor in the added costs for continuing education, updates, and equipment maintenance. Still, I love the CEREC system and am happy I can offer it to my patients.

Another futuristic-sounding technology that dentists are starting to embrace is the use of lasers in the dental practice. Lasers can be used to treat periodontal disease and can even remove decay from a tooth without having to numb a patient. The biggest hindrance to the use of lasers in a dental practice is the cost. They're high tech, super fancy, and very expensive, so they're not universally used yet. But the technology is there, and I think the more we can learn and explore, as time goes on they will become more affordable and mainstream. I can envision that in fifteen years, it will be common for dentists to use a laser to prepare a tooth and install a permanent crown without using an anesthetic. Laser dentistry may sound like science fiction, but I think it's going to be the next thing incorporated into mainstream dentistry.

Guided surgery is another modern aspect of dentistry that I believe will enter the mainstream as well. All the surgeries done at my practice are guided surgeries, and it's a meticulous process that yields the best results. The first thing I do is take an impression of my patient's teeth so I have an analog (or nondigital) version of the area we are going to work on. Then my surgeon does a cone beam scan to create a 3D image of the patient's mouth. The cone beam scan is a special kind of X-ray that uses a device that rotates around the head in a complete 360-degree path, producing a large number of images and allowing the creation of a 3D picture of the teeth, soft tissues, nerve pathways, and bone. The cone beam scan sounds kind of scary, but it's really not. It takes less than a minute and causes absolutely no discomfort. Once that's completed, the surgeon, the lab technician, and I get together and have a meeting where we determine precisely where we want to put the implants so they're in the best bone and they're angled just perfectly to ensure the strongest survival rate. This gives me exactly the access I need to position the implants. My lab technician actually makes a series of guides so we know the perfect location, orientation, and angulation for the implants. It's a remarkable procedure, and there is a lot of planning on the front end, especially for complicated or hybrid cases. We plan for every contingency, so there are no surprises, and mishaps are extremely rare.

Since I'm talking about the future of dentistry, I would like to say a few words about infection control in the dental office, because at this point we're using some pretty futuristic methods of protection at our practice. Dentists have been wearing personal protective devices like gloves and masks for many years and have very high standards for safety in the dental office. Equipment is cleaned ultrasonically and sterilized before it ever touches a patient's mouth. At many practices, including my own, we've been using eye and body protection in addition to gloves and masks even before the pandemic hit. When COVID-19 appeared, we had to increase the protection level of the masks we use to guard against aerosols, and almost every dentist I know has installed an advanced air filtration system that will filter out 99.97 percent of airborne organisms.

In my office, the air cycles six times an hour in all the rooms so that anything airborne won't have a chance to float around and cause trouble. We've also got new suction techniques and tools that we put right into the patient's mouth so that any aerosol we create is suctioned up right away. It doesn't even have a chance to get into the air. Safety is the number one priority, but unfortunately there are going to be dental offices that just can't survive because of the increased costs of the sophisticated protection. We are all about protecting both the patients and our staff from any illness, and we're confident we are doing just that. Patients need not worry about their health when they come in for a visit. Between the new filtering equipment, the better personal protective gear, and the protocols put in place, you're going to be safe, and so are we.

I hope I've given you reason to be as excited about the future of dentistry as I am. Even someone who doesn't work in the profession has to admire the awesome technology that has changed dentistry, especially over the past few decades: 3D imaging for diagnostics, the CEREC system for one-visit reconstruction, the space-age materials used to recreate natural teeth. Technological innovations have taken dentistry to a whole new level, and what will be available in the future seems limited only by the imaginations of the researchers. Many of these advances have improved the patient experience exponentially, and it's my hope that a day will come when not one single patient will avoid the dentist because they are afraid.

Technological innovations have taken dentistry to a whole new level, and what will be available in the future seems limited only by the imaginations of the researchers.

If we can get past the hurdles and get the patients into the office, I think many of them will be surprised to find a completely different environment than they might have seen years ago. In many private dental practices these days, patients can expect to find calm surroundings, state-of-the-art technology, and a highly trained staff, which together make for an all-around positive experience.

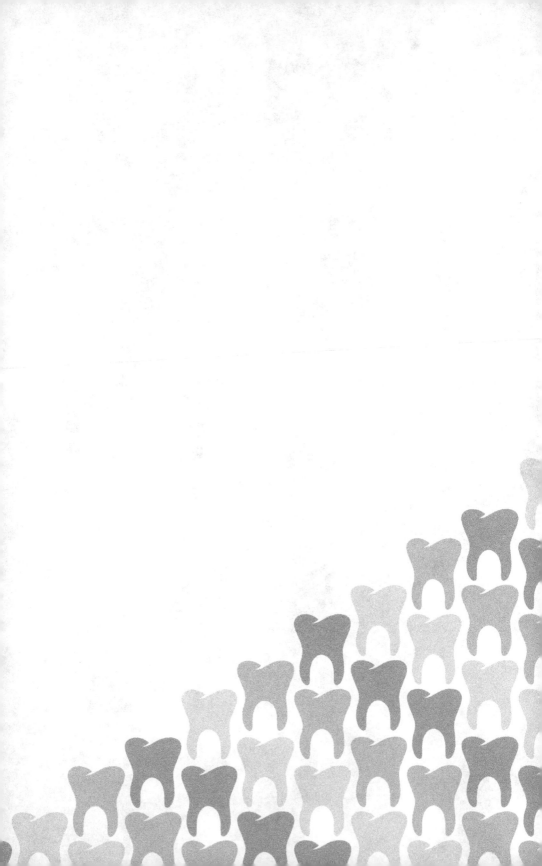

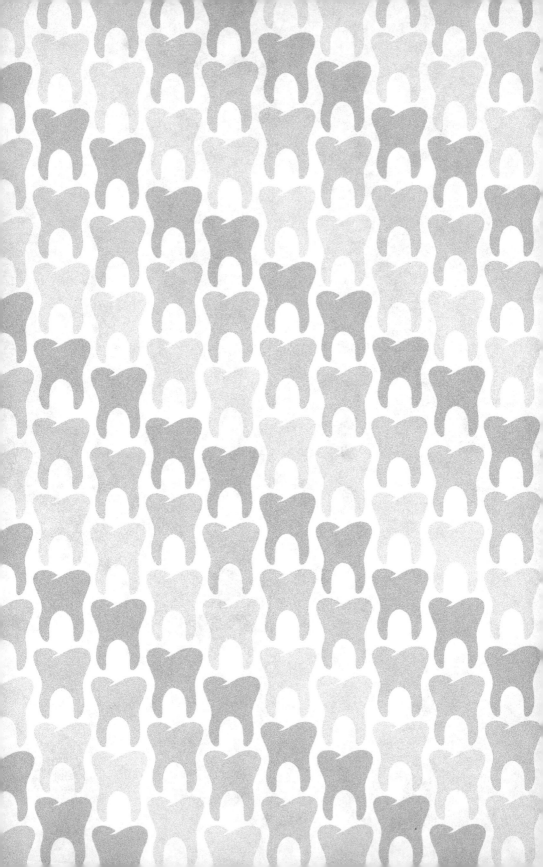

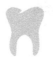

Dental Armamentarium

The tools available for oral healthcare in our modern world are fantastic, and I'd like to give you my recommendations for your own home armamentarium.

- **Toothbrush**. Electric toothbrushes are ideal. They're able to get into difficult-to-reach places, and their rotating, vibrating heads do a wonderful job. If you prefer a regular toothbrush, make sure it has soft bristles. Sorry to shout, but NO HARD BRISTLES! They can damage gum tissue, enamel, and root surfaces.

- **Toothpaste**. Choose a fluoridated toothpaste, and avoid brands with extreme bleaching properties, as they can cause scratches and staining.

- **Floss**. Regular, old-fashioned floss is fine. Floss holders and floss picks make the job even easier.

- **Tissue Stimulators**. These are great to use, but go easy. Some have a rubber tip; others have a small brush.

- **Mouth Rinse**. Choose an alcohol-free therapeutic mouthwash with an antimicrobial agent such as cetylpyridinium chloride (CPC).

- **Water Flosser**. These are unbeatable for getting into all the nooks and crannies to blast out bacteria and any leftover bits of food.

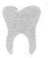

ABOUT THE AUTHOR

B rett Langston is the owner and head prosthodontist at Dental Implant and Aesthetic Specialists, a comprehensive, full-service dental practice located in Brookhaven, Georgia. Dr. Langston completed his prosthodontic residency in 2009 at the United States Healthcare Residency at Fort Gordon, Georgia, after graduating from the Medical College of Georgia in 2005 with his dental degree. Dr. Langston attended college at Saint Peter's University in New Jersey on a full-ride swimming/academic scholarship.

Dr. Langston lives in Dunwoody with his extraordinary wife, Lyndsay, who is a practicing periodontist and the owner of PerioAtlanta. They have three children—Alexis, Bella, and Knox—and they enjoy spending time together playing sports and video games. Their Catholic faith plays a huge role in the love they share and brings them great joy.

Dr. Langston is an avid learner and is a member of multiple study clubs and dental societies, such as the prestigious Thomas P. Hinman Dental Society. He enjoys staying abreast of the newest technological advancements in dentistry and is always looking for ways to improve his patients' experience and quality of care.

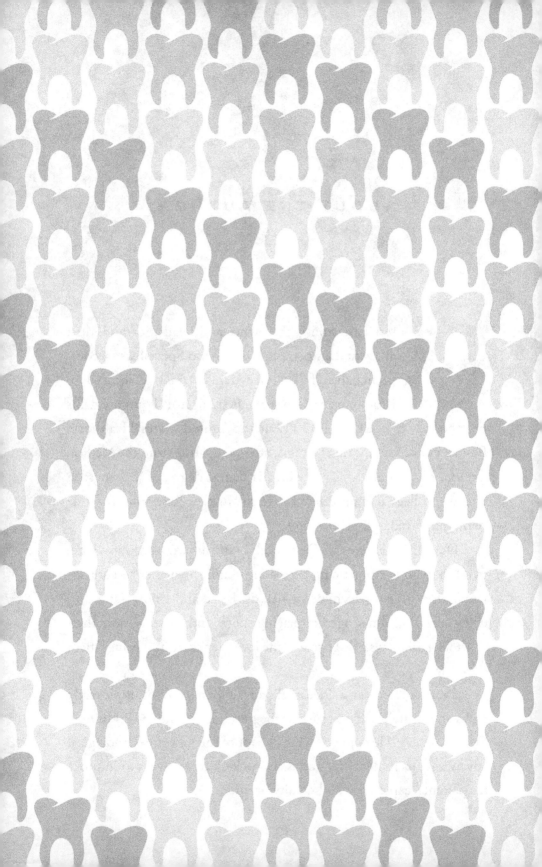

CPSIA information can be obtained
at www.ICGtesting.com
Printed in the USA
JSHW021351020623
42636JS00001B/12

9 781642 257656